Understanding the Aging Patient

Patricia A. Hess, R.N., M.S.

Assistant Professor of Nursing
San Francisco State University
San Francisco, California

with

Candra Day

Professional Writer
in association with
Textbooks Unlimited, Inc.
San Francisco, California

The Robert J. Brady Company
A Prentice - Hall Company
Bowie, Maryland 20715

Understanding the Aging Patient
First Edition

Executive Producer: Albert A. Belskie
Text Design/Production Editor: Kathye Long
Art Director/Illustrator: Don Sellers

Library of Congress Cataloging in Publication Data

Hess, Patricia A. 1938–
Understanding the aging patient.

1. Geriatric nursing. 2. Aged—Psychology.
3. Geriatrics. 4. Aging. I. Day, Candra,
1948– joint author. II. Title
RC954.H43 618.9'7 77–2596

ISBN 0–87618–733–5

Prentice-Hall International, Inc., London
Prentice-Hall of Australia, Pty., Ltd., Sydney
Prentice-Hall of India Private Limited, New Delhi
Prentice-Hall of Japan, Inc., Tokyo
Prentice-Hall of Southeast Asia (Pte.) Ltd., Singapore
Whitehall Books Limited, Wellington, New Zealand

Printed in the United States of America

77 78 79 80 81 82 83 10 9 8 7 6 5 4 3 2 1

Contents

Preface

In recent years geriatric nursing has witnessed two fundamental changes. First, the notion that old age is characterized by inevitable and irreversible degeneration, requiring medical care primarily for maintenance and comfort, is being replaced by a new attitude. We now are finding that old people often respond well to treatment, particularly if it is geared to their special needs. Second, a new need is felt for in-service training in the field of geriatrics to familiarize working nurses with recent developments in gerontology. These two trends comprise the orientation of this book.

We propose to approach the subject of geriatric nursing holistically, on the premise that social and psychic factors are intimately linked to physical disorders. This is particularly crucial among the aged. We will focus on multidimensional treatment that is based on an understanding of the interaction of multiple systems in geriatric patients.

The book is divided into three sections. Section I focuses on our present knowledge of normal aging and the implications of this knowledge for nursing care. Section II is devoted to the common diseases of old age, with special attention to nursing care for communication and mental disorders. Section III explores restorative geriatric nursing, including planning for continuity of care. This format enables us to review the major areas of the field in a positive way, beginning with an understanding of normal aging and concluding with an emphasis on restorative nursing practice.

We have attempted to highlight the rewards of geriatric nursing. A doctor told me recently about an elderly woman who was semicomatose most of the time. Occasionally, though, the old lady had a few hours of complete clarity. Then, she was so full of appreciation and enjoyment of life that everyone near her was enlivened. The doctor said that this lady had helped her to understand the fragility of life. "She reminded us of that treasure, the spark of life."

This book is intended to help nurses provide outstanding care for their geriatric patients. The need for such a book is clear: Geriatrics is usually studied only minimally in nursing schools. The elderly population is increasing both absolutely and relatively in the United States and comes into increasing contact with the medical profession, usually posing special problems for nursing care. Particularly since many elderly patients are isolated from other community sources of support, nurses recognize a responsibility to understand and treat the whole individual.

The scope of the field of geriatrics is overwhelming. This book is only an introduction, and we hope it will be a stimulus to further exploration of the kinds of care available for older people.

Introduction

Nursing the older patient is a highly creative process. Knowledge, alertness, and concern must be joined with imagination, warmth, patience, and perseverance in caring for the elderly. With these tools, the nurse creates a therapeutic environment, and helps to direct the process of healing.

In this book the importance of a creative approach is emphasized. All the evidence indicates that the first step in geriatric nursing is a positive attitude about old age. We have seen that social and cultural conditions of old age can directly contribute to disease. The nurse's initial act is to dispel the pervasive negative assumptions concerning the aged.

Current knowledge about the dynamics of normal aging emphasizes both the individuality of each old person and the typical lack of tolerance to stress in all its forms. This awareness is crucial to restorative nursing; it leads to a personal, unique relationship, sensitive to the dynamics of many factors. We hope, in addition, that this book enables the nurse to differentiate between the normal effects of aging and pathologic conditions.

Restorative nursing of the elderly is based on aggressive practice and the continual assessment of the interplay of physical, emotional, and social factors. The evidence strongly suggests that older patients often respond well to treatment, especially when the nurse pursues an individualized care plan and is alert to danger signs. A great deal of new information about gerontology is now available, and much success can be achieved in the care of the elderly.

A good illustration of this creative nursing practice is the care of a person with aphasia. Imagination and patience are what is wanted, since such diverse techniques as singing may help, memorization may help, graphics may help, and any way the nurse can find to alleviate anxiety will surely help. The byword is *try it*!

Mental disorders also call for this kind of care. Reality orientation and remotivation programs have met with considerable success. Establishing a warm, therapeutic relationship with a patient will diminish the loneliness and isolation that often lead to physical breakdown. Again, the theme is *try it*!

We have illustrated the importance of continuity of care to the elderly and the key role of the nurse in this service. This facet of caregiving depends as well on imaginative and informed problem-solving.

We have spoken earlier about the satisfactions of geriatric nursing, but not enough has yet been said about the fun of working with older people. It is a joy to free oneself from the myths about old age and to see old age as a promising part of life, for oneself as well as for others. It is like throwing off blinders. And it is a great and lasting pleasure to work with older people who have seen much and enjoyed much, and have survived to pass it on. It is exciting to see the world—and ourselves—through their experienced eyes, though we may often feel like young squirts with a lot to learn. There are often plenty of jokes, for older people take the time for a good laugh. Finally, working closely with older people brings with it a heightened sense of the preciousness and flow of life. Geriatric nursing can enable the older individual—and the nurse—to lead a more meaningful life.

Acknowledgments

We wish to thank Mary Thomas, Faith Bartlett, Dolores Tyberg, and Charlotte Offhouse, nurses all, for sharing their insights and expertise so generously and for transmitting the satisfactions they have found in working with older people.

Understanding the Aging Patient

I

Normal Aging

Chapter 1

A Philosophy of Aging for Geriatric Nursing

Unless we can create a world which offers the possibility of aging with grace, honor, and meaningfulness, no one can look forward to the future.

—Seymour Halleck[1]

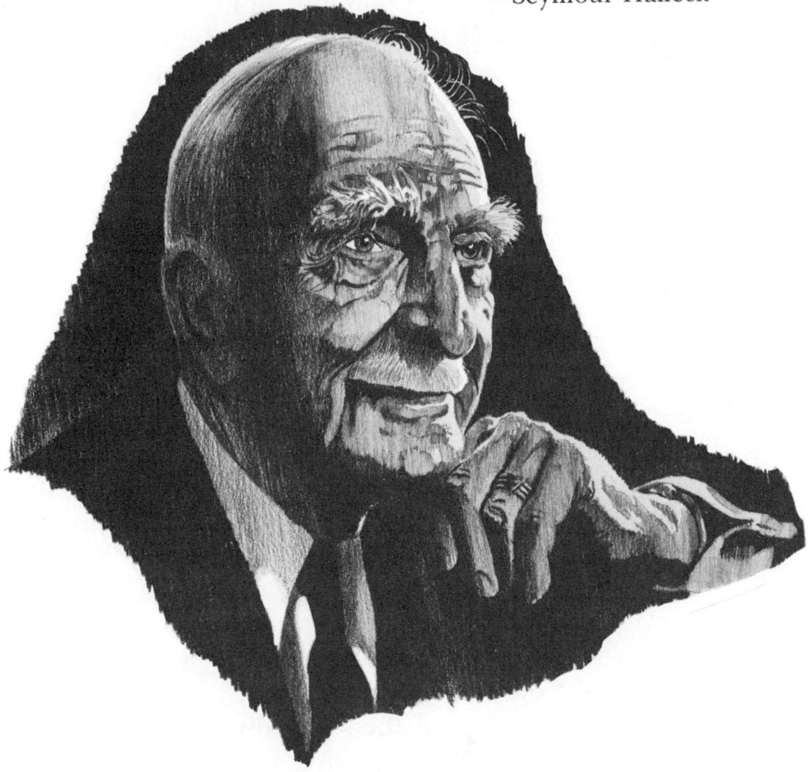

THE PROSPECTS OF OLD AGE

In essence, Halleck's statement is what geriatric nursing is all about: the creation, through care, of a world for our elderly patients that offers grace, honor, and meaningfulness for both their living and their dying. Yet it is an impossible task unless we know the dynamics of aging and understand the special needs of the older patient—who the aged are, how they live, and what guidelines can be defined for nursing care.

Who Are the Aged?

Our society usually delineates old age as the period of life after age 65. Although chronological age is a convenient way of categorizing people, it is frequently an inaccurate indicator of an individual's physical or mental status. Chronological age does not provide much useful evidence about human beings.[2]

There are more than 22 million Americans over 65; more than one million over 85; more than 100,000 over 100 years of age.[2] Our population of elderly people has risen dramatically in the last century, and continues to increase in proportion to the rest of the population as well as in total numbers. Of these, over 95% live in the community, not in institutions, 86% are able to go out without difficulty, and only 2.3% are bedfast.[3] Health professionals generally come into contact with people who are ill and need help, and may lose sight of how many others are living successfully at home.

Older women outnumber older men. Approximately one in five live in poor households, and at least half have not completed 8 years of formal education.[4] A larger proportion of older people needs medical care and has chronic diseases more often than younger people, and the older people require more care for their ills.

Statistics may help to establish a norm, but of course they shed little light on the circumstances of any individual. Practitioners are well aware of the social diversity—ethnic, educational, and financial—of people over 65.

Historical factors influence the consciousness of each generation, and it is helpful to acknowledge the historical experience of our present generation of elderly. Born near the turn of the century when "survival of the fittest" was a popular social theory, and the Protestant ethic of hard work and self-sacrifice was the dominant religious influence in America, many of these people resist the emerging national acceptance of responsibility for all citizens. They may find the surcease of work with retirement extremely difficult and interpret economic problems as personal failure. Many older people feel ambivalent about Social Security and Medicare, and their lifetime experience with rapid growth of industrialization and automation may increase their feelings of uselessness and complicate their adjustment to present social circumstances.

In addition, many older Americans are foreign-born and retain a cultural identity with their homeland. Their past experience and system of belief are often difficult for younger Americans to understand.

How Do They Live?

Prevailing cultural attitudes lead many Americans to believe that the happy, successfully functioning older people they know are exceptional. Successful old age is actually the rule rather than the exception. In spite of a doleful lack of social support, old age is for many a period of discovery and satisfaction. Health professionals and the communications media tend to overemphasize illness and problems in later life and ignore the rewards of longevity.

There is an urgent need to find a balance between concentration on pathologic conditions and positive orientation toward the qualities of aging. It is often hard to know whether physiological aging processes are contributing to the negative stereotypes of old age or the stereotypes derive, instead, from a disuse of mind and body forced upon the elderly by our cultural attitudes. Frequently, it is not the normal biological changes but their subsequent effects on self-regard that have the greatest impact on the individual.[5] Health professionals have a responsibility to dispel stereotypes of decrepitude and correct negative attitudes about old age.

The elderly person has a unique set of tasks to do that are commensurate with the capacities of the aging. The old person must be as flexible as the young to promote and maintain health.

There are four major developmental tasks of old age:

To clarify, deepen, and find use for a lifetime of experience;
To conserve strength and resources;
To adjust to changes and losses; and
To enjoy the achievement of being "a completed human being.[2]

The elderly person has to learn to relinquish power and some activities. In so doing, he often develops a self-transcendent philosophy of life that is important both for himself and for others.[6] The aged often savor life intensely, and are able to relish the joy of daily living. Old age is often a time to *be* instead of *do,* and to pursue self-fulfillment and self-actualization.[3] For the elderly who wish to leave a legacy to coming generations, this capacity for enjoying life is a most valuable one.

Other common positive qualities of old age are increased wisdom and judgment, as well as a more stable sense of values gained through years of experience. Later life is also characterized by decreased responsibilities; the elderly are not expected to work, and certain economic benefits may accrue to them. The aged frequently do not fear death and acquire a heightened degree of serenity toward life's changes.[3] All these qualities vary, of course, from individual to individual, but they surely deserve at least as much attention as illness and loss of certain capacities.

Implications for Nursing Care

1. Geriatric nursing emphasizes the participation of the patient in all phases of the care-giving process.
2. Since the elderly population is so diversified, nurses need an acute awareness of how each person has lived in the past, what are the priorities and values of each one, and what are the future hopes of each. To give care, the nurse needs to know how the patient thinks and feels, as good intentions alone will not help.
3. In the care of the elderly patient in an institutional setting, it is imperative that the impact of institutional isolation be

recognized. Separated from family, meaningful social contact, and familiar surroundings, the aged patient often feels severe emotional deprivation. Interventions to ease that sense of isolation are extremely important.

4. Personal involvement is necessary in geriatric nursing, especially in a long-term setting. It is beneficial for both patient and nurse in any setting. Involvement means that the patient's unique needs will be understood and acted upon. It means that care will be personalized and sensitive. For the nurse, listening and learning often reveals the promise of aging. Her work is rewarded by a self-discovery of her own possible future.

STANDARDS OF CARE

The American Nurses' Association has formulated a set of standards for geriatric nursing based on our present knowledge of gerontology.[7] These standards are basic reference points for giving quality care to the aged patient.

Standard I

The nurse demonstrates an appreciation of the heritage, values and wisdom of older persons.

The nurse has some understanding of the social and historical factors that influence the behavior and values of older people. This appreciation enables her to respect the aged patient, to nurture self-respect, and to enrich her own life. Some important social factors in aging are discussed in Chapter 2.

Standard II

The nurse seeks to resolve her conflicting attitudes regarding aging, death, and dependency so that she can assist older persons and their relatives to maintain life with dignity and comfort until death ensues.

Individualized care and respect for dignity help to make the sick role for the elderly easier to bear. The nurse cannot provide such care without an awareness of her own feelings. In

Chapter 7 the subject of nursing care for the dying patient is explored.

Standard III

The nurse observes and interprets minimal as well as gross signs and symptoms associated with both normal aging and pathologic changes and institutes appropriate nursing measures.

The better portion of this book is designed to help nurses with this process of assessment and intervention. The normal physiological changes of aging are discussed in Chapter 3; the management of the most common pathologic states, Chapter 4; and highlights of the fundamentals of restorative nursing for the aged, Chapter 8. Nurses need to be able to distinguish between normal aging and pathologic changes.

Standard IV

The nurse differentiates between pathologic social behavior and the usual life style of each aged individual.

These distinctions are often difficult to draw. Is a patient's withdrawal a manifestation of the right for privacy or is it a sign of illness and/or depression? Are nurses imposing irrelevant personal judgments on a patient's unusual behavior? Mental disorders in later life are the subject of Chapter 6. We hope the discussion will help the nurse to make correct decisions in questions of this kind.

Standard V

The nurse supports and promotes normal physiologic functioning of the older person.

The emphasis here is on the nurse's role in selecting adequate food, encouraging health-promoting exercise and habit patterns, proper skin care, and in supporting independent functioning. Information in Chapter 8 will help the nurse to pursue these goals.

Standard VI

The nurse protects aged persons from injury, infection, and excessive stress and supports them through the multiplicity of stressful experiences to which they are subjected.

The aged have a decreased capacity to cope with stress, and a higher incidence of stressful experiences. The nurse uses appropriate interventions to prevent or alleviate stress and to enhance the patient's coping ability. Stress in the normal aging process is discussed in some detail in Chapters 2 and 3, and nursing measures are suggested throughout the book.

Standard VII

The nurse employs a variety of methods to promote effective communication and social interaction of aged persons with individuals, family, and other groups.

Chapter 5 is concerned with communication disorders of blindness, deafness, and aphasia. It offers some suggestions for nursing actions to facilitate communication and social interaction. Therapeutic relationships, both one-to-one and in groups, are discussed in Chapter 8.

Standard VIII

The nurse and the older person together design, change, or adapt the physical and psychosocial environment to meet that person's needs within the limits imposed by the situation.

In an institutional setting, the nurse's responsibility includes providing an optimal environment for the patient's well-being. The nurse also plans for continuity of care to help the patient adapt his home environment to meet his changing needs. Some key principles of continuity of care are presented in Chapter 9.

Standard IX

The nurse assists older persons to obtain and utilize devices that help them attain a higher level of functioning and ensures that these devices are kept in good working order by the appropriate persons or agencies.

Devices such as wheelchairs, walkers, hearing aids, and other prostheses are essential supportive measures to facilitate functioning. A defective device may be dangerous. Nurses need to be familiar with resources for obtaining and maintaining these devices. The chapter on continuity of care (Chapter 9) includes some ideas for possible resources.

To keep the book succinct, we have included only a few case histories. Your own experience as a nurse adds the person and personality of the elderly individual. The book is not a comprehensive review of the field. We are only trying to convey the "state of the art" of geriatric nursing, and to elucidate the basic concepts of modern gerontologic nursing.

THE REWARDS OF GERIATRIC NURSING

Geriatric nursing has begun to emerge as a gratifying career in the last 10 years, after having been one of the most unpopular nursing specialties in the past. Geriatric nurses very frequently say that they love their work, and would not change to any other field.[8,9] It is a challenging job, demanding a wide range of clinical expertise as well as uncommon alertness and sensitivity, and the satisfactions in doing such a difficult and important task are great.

The aged need the opportunity to tell of their lives, and the young need the opportunity to listen. Geriatric nursing affords the nurse a chance to learn from the elderly, and in turn to provide support and recognition.

Now is a turning point for nurses and older people both, an opportunity for mutual enlightenment. There is still a great deal to learn about aging, but what is now known is a "good beginning."

> A great deal of talent is lost in the world from want of little courage. Every day sends to their graves obscure men whom timidity prevented from making a first effort: who, if they could have been induced to begin, would have in all probability gone great lengths in the career of same. The fact is that to do anything in the world worth doing, we must not stand back shiver-

ing and thinking of the cold and danger but jump in and scramble through as well as we can.

—Richard Cardinal Cushing[10]

REFERENCES

[1]Halleck, S.: In *Nursing and the Aged*. Edited by I.M. Burnside. New York: McGraw-Hill, 1976.

[2]Butler, R.N., and Lewis, M.I.: *Aging and Mental Health.* St. Louis: C.V. Mosby Co., 1973.

[3]Hayter, J.: Positive Aspects of Aging. *J. Gerontol. Nurs*. 2:19, 1976.

[4]Weg, R.: The aged: Who, where, how well. Ethel Andrus Percy Gerontological Center, University of Southern California, Los Angeles, 1975.

[5]Curtin, S.R.: *Nobody Ever Died of Old Age.* Boston: Little, Brown & Co., 1972.

[6]Ebersole, P.: "Developmental Tasks in Late Life." In *Nursing and the Aged.* Edited by I.M. Burnside. New York: McGraw-Hill, 1976.

[7]Executive Committee and the Standards Committee of the Division on Geriatric Nursing Practice: *Standards for Geriatric Nursing.* American Nurses' Association, Kansas City, Mo. 1973. (Though these standards were updated in 1976, the authors felt it was more fitting for their purposes to use the 1973 standards.)

[8]Boward, M.E.: Gerontological nursing is not boring or depressing. *J. Gerontol. Nurs.* 1:28, 1975.

[9]Thomas, Mary R.N., B.S.N., Director of Nursing, Marin Convalescent Hospital, personal communication, March 1976, Tiburon, Calif.

[10]Cushing, R.: In *Nursing and the Aged.* Edited by I.M. Burnside. New York: McGraw-Hill, 1976.

SUGGESTED READING

Philibert, M.: Philosophy of aging: Implications for nursing. In *Nursing and the Aged*. Edited by I.M. Burnside. New York: McGraw-Hill, 1976.

Chapter 2

The Psychosocial Dynamics of Aging

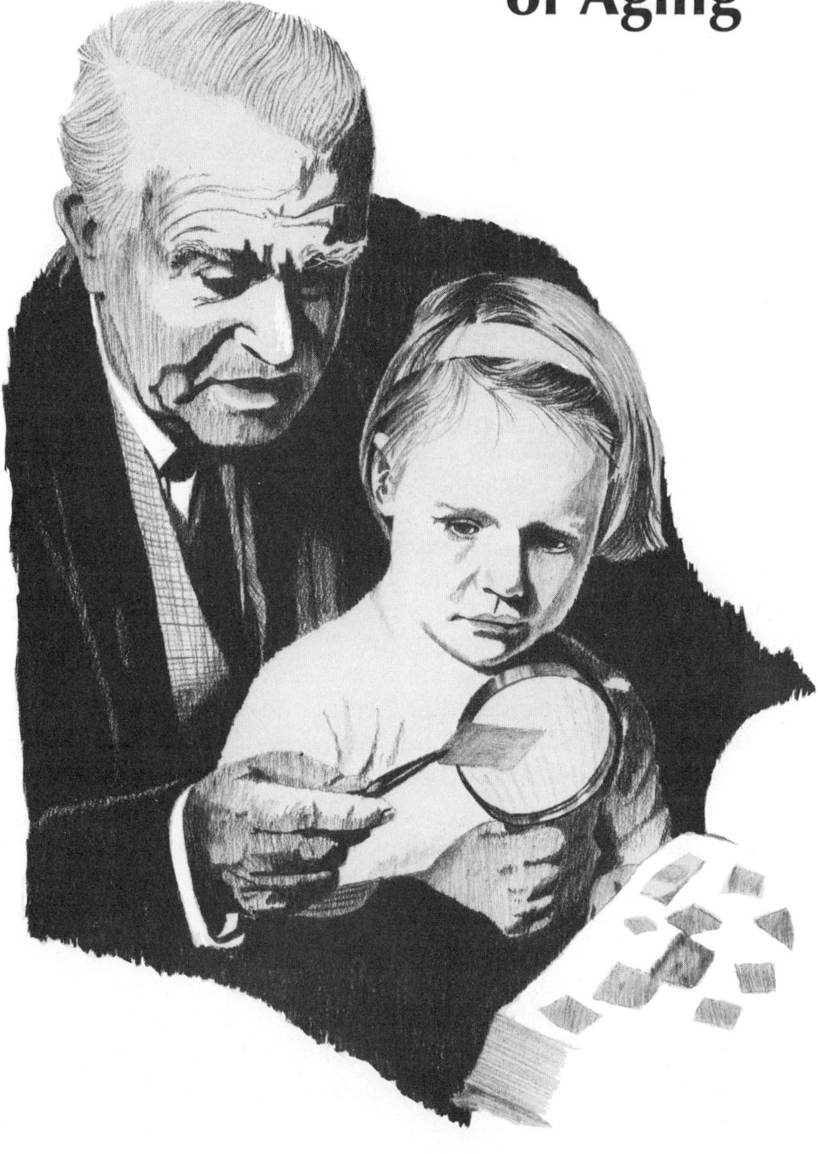

Normal old age is a period of enormous learning and growth. Outwardly, in relationships with other people, the older person learns to adapt to the circumstances of old age. The elderly often meet this challenge with a degree of wit, imagination, and strength of spirit that can tax the resources of younger people. Inwardly, they summon a lifetime's accumulation of experience for review and integration. This life review process may bring with it the inner rewards of the examined life.

All the preparation of a lifetime is a resource for growth in old age. There is an uninterrupted continuity from youth to age. The challenges of old age are familiar to other ages as well, and each individual has unique, long-established patterns of behavior.

People who were conservative and cautious as youths usually become conservative elders; lifelong rebels become old rebels. A case in point:

> January 1972 found Jeannette Rankin of Missoula, Montana, 91, lifelong pacifist and activist, the first woman to win membership in the U.S. House of Representatives, living in a house with a dirt floor in her living room. She gave her money to the peace movement. She demonstrated what Emerson said of Thoreau, that he made himself rich by making his wants few. In 1968, at 87, she led the Jeannette Rankin Brigade of 5,000 women to Washington to protest the Vietnam War. She was quoted (*New York Times,* January 1972) as saying that if she had her life to relive, "I'd be nastier."[1]

A most striking consequence of the aging process is the intensification of individuality. A group of 16-year-olds is noticeably more homogeneous than a group of 40-year-olds, and individualization continues in the later years. Recent longitudinal studies (especially Neugarten's[2]) emphasize great individual differences among the aged above all other findings.

What does this mean? For one thing, it means that chronological age is a poor indication of a person's characteristics. It means that individualities are more important than commonalities in understanding the aged. It further means that our cultural tendency to arbitrarily categorize the elderly runs counter to what we actually know about the aging process.

This conflict between cultural attitudes and the realities of old age profoundly affects the psychosocial process of aging in America.

It is impossible to isolate normal aging from its milieu, and in this culture, we do not like or respect old people. The first steps for care-giving are recognizing and understanding these attitudes and freeing ourselves from their constraint.

OUR SOCIAL MYTHS OF AGING

The norm in our society is a general—almost phobic—dislike of aging, a focus on illness, and a disregard for healthy old people. Rarely will you find a person who looks forward enthusiastically to old age, and yet this pervasive attitude is based on fictions rather than facts. Most of our images of old age come from social workers, who know only the poor and isolated, or physicians, who know only the ill. They do not reflect the typical.

Medical science has mirrored these social attitudes: In the past, *decline* of the individual was the key concept and *neglect,* the major treatment. The sick role is oftentimes more socially acceptable than health for the elderly. It is expected and accepted. Now, however, understanding is growing that this approach is intolerable. Neglect, indeed, encourages decline, but restorative nursing care usually leads to improvement and successes. The breakthroughs in geriatric nursing begin with an understanding of these myths and their probabilities for becoming self-fulfilling.

Ageism, the prejudice against age, is a way of categorizing old people and not allowing them to be unique. We separate ourselves from them and relegate them to an inferior status. Restorative nursing discards the myths and the segregation to which they lead.

Part of this cultural mythology is a series of common assumptions about the elderly as a group. These assumptions are misleading, and often harmful:

The myth of chronological age. Chronological age is not a reliable indicator of aging. It is more accurate to say that "you're as old as you feel" than to rely on chronological age as a dependable description of an elderly person. Our social method of arbitrarily typing people as old at 65 (for retirement, social security, etc.) causes much frustration and hardship.

The senility myth. Senility is a term used far too loosely by both medical and lay people, but it is not a part of normal aging. Many emotional reactions such as depression, grief, and anxiety are often labeled as senile, and therefore untreatable. The myth of senility itself causes anxiety among the elderly.

The tranquility myth. The myth that aging is associated with tranquility perpetuates the picture of the serene, idyllic grandma (reminiscent of the myth of "happy, jolly black folks") without recognition of the many challenges of old age.

The myth of unproductivity. Older people are often assumed to be disinterested in active lives. In the absence of disease, the elderly usually continue their involvement in the community. This question of disengagement will be further discussed later in this chapter.

The myth of resistance to change. Resistance to change is not inherent in aging, but rather depends on lifelong personality patterns. Socioeconomic pressures may also contribute to conservatism.

The myth of taboos. Sexuality is commonly discouraged or ignored in later life, although sex remains important. Sexuality and self-esteem are closely related, and sexuality should be encouraged to preserve sexual capacities.

The myth of unhappy old age. Probably the most insidious myth of all is that old age is usually unpleasant. Numerous studies have shown that age is a poor indicator of the differences between people. It is a particularly harmful belief because it is so often self-fulfilling. As a result of social neglect, old people may find themselves lonely, ill, and isolated. Our cultural emphasis on productivity and achievement and our exclusion of death from life often lead us to see old people as "failing." Old age can be—and often is—a satisfying and enriching time. A national survey indicates that three-fourths of the elderly are satisfied or very satisfied with life after retirement. Most consider themselves to be in good health.[2]

SOCIAL DEMOGRAPHY OF THE ELDERLY

The social facts about the elderly belie the attitude of "failing" old age. Ninety-five percent of people over 65 live successfully in the community—in rural areas or central cities. Only 5% are institutionalized. The number and proportion of the aged is a new and fast-growing phenomenon in our society. Between 1960 and 1974, the number of people aged 65–74 increased 23%; the number over 75 increased 49%. This is in contrast to an 11.5% increase in people under 45. Today, every tenth American is over 65.

Income. Social statistics, however, reveal the many ways in which our attitudes affect the lives of the elderly. It is estimated that, because of poverty, 30% live in substandard housing. In 1971, half of the elderly lived on less than $75 a week, and one-fourth had annual incomes under $1,872. (This group includes both the lifelong poor and the newly poor.) The remaining one-fourth had annual incomes over $9,000. Of this income, 29% is earned, and the rest derives from retirement plans and social security benefits. Many of the elderly are isolated economically as well as socially.

Marital status. There are 90 men to every 100 women over 65. Most men are married; most women are widows. Each year, the number of older men who marry is more than twice the number of older women who do so, despite the greater number of women. This means that there is a large number of widows. The taboo against sexuality in later life makes the lot of elderly women unnecessarily difficult.

Special concerns. Racism affects the elderly as well as the young. Black men die younger than white men; they are more often unmarried. Some kind of income-maintenance plan is urgently needed. There is a need also for more racially mixed professional services to provide alternate care methods more appropriate to minority groups. Sexism also continues in old age; Butler and Lewis call the mistreatment of old women a "national habit."[1]

The situation of the rural aged is significantly different from that of the urban aged. They are able to work longer, and are, therefore, usually better off financially. They still need to adapt to many changes in living situations.

Religion. There is some indication of heightened inner religious feeling among the elderly, but there is little change of interest in established religion. Most people continue their earlier patterns.

THE PSYCHOSOCIAL PROCESS OF AGING

These statistics about the elderly do not evoke a living picture of the social life of our old people, but they do offer a basis upon which to view the dynamic psychosocial process of old age. What is the day-by-day experience of the 22 million older people in the United States?

Imagine yourself old (if you are not) and wend your way through the social maze of aging. Comtemplate the accomplishments of the elderly:

> *You are 65, healthy and active. Retirement from your job of 20 years is compulsory. It means a freedom and leisure you have long dreamed of, and yet, when the day arrives, you discover that the work habit is hard to break. What are you going to do this week? Next week? You begin to realize that you will have to learn a whole new way of life. . . .*

For some, retirement is liberation; for others, it constitutes a profound psychological crisis. Consider these stories:

> When Alice Langhorn retired as manager of a Chicago clothing store, she said: "Getting up late for breakfast. No pell-mell rush to work. No customers or board of directors to hound me. What a life it's going to be." Months later, she began to feel very restless. She missed her friends from work, and began to feel out of things. Time stretched out interminably, and she was trou-

bled by spells of depression. "You've got to know how to retire," she concluded. "And I guess I wasn't prepared for it."[3]

An article in the Nov. 25, 1975, *San Francisco Chronicle* reports on two women: Helen Salz, 92, a retired educator and founder of a well-known school is now a respected painter and an active civil libertarian. Flora Arnstein, 90, a retired teacher, is now a poet and a teacher of poetry. Here is one of Mrs. Arnstein's recent poems:

For M.E.T.

You are unanswerable:
Filament of summer,
A shell whorl,
A submerged footprint
In the outdrifting tide,
A grape vine grappling,
Tree, twigs, temples . . .
Because of shade and shadow,
Because of no promises,
Because in this inch of time
You begrudge no breath,
Because before you I am a pilgrim
Who worships and departs,
His cup empty, but with a ringing of bells.

"I'm going crazy with nothing to do. . . . But give me some job I can do."

—Retired foreman of a manufacturing company

When retirement is felt to be a great loss, it may lead to physiological disease. Even when it is seen as an opportunity for freedom, it requires *change* and learning.

Another hurdle of old age, unconnected to any specific year, is adjustment to a decrease in physical energy and strength.

Gradually, over the years, you find you cannot move as quickly as you used to. You tire more readily, and fear somewhat for your health. You notice–much to your dismay–that your hearing or vision is poorer.

Or you may develop a chronic illness with severe limitations. You have to adjust your patterns of living. You may have to cope with hospitalization.

Or your spouse may become ill, and require constant nursing. He may also become increasingly anxious and irritable.

All these circumstances demand continuous adjustment and creative problem-solving.

Loss is a common predicament of old age. The old often encounter financial losses and loss of prestige and status as well as physical losses. People of all ages suffer these losses occasionally, but the elderly almost always experience some loss, and sometimes multiple losses occur simultaneously. These challenge a person's coping capacities, but no loss is so difficult as the death of a husband or wife, or of loved friends or children.

How would you respond to this crisis? Through grief, as we all do. As St. Augustine wrote in his confessions:

> A huge wave of sorrow flooded my heart and flowed outward in tears. . . . What, then, was it which caused grievous pain within me, if not the fresh wound arising from the sudden breaking of a very sweet and cherished habit of living together?

Grief follows a predictable pattern. It begins with a feeling of numbness and the inability to accept the loss. Then shock and great distress follow, and often feelings of guilt, anger, and uncontrollable irritability.

Grief is a long and painful process. Although *acute* grief may last only a month, the feelings persist normally for as long as a year, and are quickly reawakened by further loss or stress. Grief brings with it a sense of unreality, of emptiness and suffocation; it may bring delusions and disorganization. It is difficult to sleep or to eat.

Yet it has a healing purpose. Grief enables one to adapt to the reality of a loss and to begin to find ways of coming to terms with new circumstance. With the elderly, the process is especially painful because it becomes increasingly difficult to find any kind of substitute for such losses. Yet most older people endure their grief, resolve it, learn from it, and carry on. A great deal of energy is expended in grief; bereavement is the single most crucial factor in predicting physical or mental breakdown.

Grief may be delayed or prolonged. It may be postponed for days or even months and may manifest itself in somatic illness or in activity rather than through mourning. Chronic grief may remain unresolved for years.

Anticipatory grief, such as a wife may experience when caring for her dying husband, is a protective device to prepare for an expected loss. It may lead to premature withdrawal from a dying loved one.

> *You–as an oldster–may encounter other feelings which are new to you, and which test your capacity to adjust. Since social interaction often becomes more limited (no work, fewer friends, less energy to get around), and since society tends to isolate you from the larger world, you may find yourself lonely.*

When senior citizens were asked about the most common mental health problems of the elderly, they mentioned loneliness more often than anything else. Family may live far away, and many find themselves living alone after years of married life.

There are several different kinds of loneliness. Nurses need to determine the specific cause or causes of loneliness to implement appropriate interventions. Loneliness may be geographical, a consequence of physical isolation. It may be caused by language barriers or by cultural isolation. It may be brought about by an individual's particular life style, or by illness and pain.

Loneliness often accompanies grief. Impending death brings loneliness to some, since many people are unable to relate to the dying. Health care requires a creative, thoughtful approach tailored to each individual. Much loneliness—especially in nursing homes—is caused by "years of neglect by a society . . . more ready to disburse funds for incarceration than for regeneration."[4] Restorative nursing reverses this process, and provides companionship and care.

Not all people who are alone are lonely. In fact, the discovery of aloneness without loneliness may be one of the victories of old age. One woman of 87 said that she was extremely lonely for her deeply loved husband for years after his death but came to realize that finally she was no longer lonely. She had made peace with her loss and was very satisfied with her life. "I'm not lonely now. That's the main thing."

There are other emotional reactions that older people often experience. The effort of meeting the tasks at hand—the adaptation to new circumstances, to disease or to death—may cause severe anxiety. In all learning, anxiety develops in proportion to the task at hand. In addition, medical professionals may induce severe anxiety—even pathologic states—through careless explanations.

Some interesting experiments have been conducted to study the impact of social changes normally associated with aging. Kastenbaum used young subjects—aged 20 to 30—but tried to simulate conditions of old age; that is, he tried to recreate the aged's "task at hand."[3] He gave his subjects a task to accomplish, and then demanded that they gradually speed up their performance until they were trying to work almost twice as fast. (The slower speed of response of many older people inspired the experiment.) He found that his subjects were unable to learn from their errors or change direction when they were required to speed up. They responded with anxiety, frustration, sometimes passive acceptance of failure, sometimes rage.[5] Older people may experience a similar sense of impotence or helplessness, responding in anger.

Unresolved grief, loneliness, guilt, or anger may lead to depression. Sometimes depression is normal and transient; at other times, it is a pathologic symptom that requires special care.

What did you feel during your imaginary aging? Sorrow? Rage? Resignation? Did you also feel the freedom that comes with retirement, or the peace that comes with understanding and acceptance? Older people experience both ends of this emotional spectrum as they "learn" to age.

Did you feel weary and empty, or did you discover sources of meaning and insight? Perhaps this is the greatest individual difference of all.

As we have seen, our general social attitudes are far from supportive of old people. In restorative nursing, the social environment becomes supportive, respectful, and understanding. What a difference this makes in the dynamics of aging!

THE FAMILY

The social environment of the elderly is not usually one of complete isolation and neglect. The family is the key source of interaction for old people, and evidence does not support the idea of oldsters abandoned by their families. Although both generations often prefer separate households, old people are not neglected. If they have children, they often live within 5 or 10 miles of at least one child; 84% live within an hour of their children, and only 7% live farther than 2 hours away.[1] Even with the high mobility of American society, geographical distance does not usually mean emotional distance. Families usually keep in close touch, and help and support one another.

Old people have an important familial role as grandparents or, increasingly, as great-grandparents.

The reports of old people indicate that being a grandparent is a joyful and satisfying role. They often take great pleasure in their grandchildren, providing companionship and guidance to them and help to the parents. The image of the stern, authoritarian grandparent is being replaced by the help-giving, modern-day grandparent, who, in our day, is often not old, but still middle-aged.

The family is not only a help-giving unit in all directions, and an avenue for interaction. It is often the vehicle through which learning and understanding is transmitted between the generations. It embodies the continuity of human life from generation to generation.

This function is beautifully illustrated in a screenplay by Dick Eribes called "I Remember the Future as Though It were Yesterday."

An elderly father is moving from his large house after his wife's death, and he and his son decide to have a garage sale of his lifetime's belongings. His son is all business, while the father wanders around examining the things as though he were another thoughtful customer. A young boy comes along, and stops to look at a bike that had once belonged to the old man's son. The boy admired the bike, and the old man, explaining that it was once his son's, gave it to him. The son was angry; he said the bicycle was worth $20. But the father had taken something out of the past and given it a future.[6] A remarkable perspective, "I Remember the Future as Though It Were Yesterday."

SOCIAL THEORIES OF AGING

Both psychologists and sociologists have presented hypotheses to explain the psychosocial process of aging, and to account for observed changes in the behavior patterns of elderly people. The field of inquiry is new and undeveloped; two of the theories are diametrically opposed. Yet nurses have found these ideas useful in caring for the elderly, insofar as they help in understanding behavior and generating respect for the complex dynamics of aging.

The Activity Theory

This orientation may be expressed as Johann Johnson, 73, did: ". . . keep active—I want to wear out, not rust out."[7] More an orientation than a strict theory, this line of thinking holds that norms and expectations do not change significantly in later life, that the individual's personality remains fairly stable with increasing age and that the major social need of the elderly is opportunities for activity to replace work and other social losses. The sources of satisfaction and self-esteem are not expected to change significantly.

The theory proposes that there is a positive relation between social activity and life satisfaction in old age and that role loss (such as in widowhood or retirement) decreases life satisfaction. There is considerable doubt whether this theory is substantiated by the available data.

Disengagement Theory

The disengagement theory holds that the aging process is seen as a mutual withdrawal—a disengaging—of the individual and society. In contrast with the activity theory, it suggests that decreased activity is the norm, and that this disengagement is satisfying both to the individual and society. It suggests that old age *is* significantly different from middle age, with new norms and expectations.

This theory has met with considerable attention, and has caused much debate. Although it is generally accepted that activity levels decrease with age, there is sharp disagreement about the meaning of this decrease and its effect on life satisfaction. Recently, the theory has been further developed by Cumming (one of the initial formulators) to include a distinction between two personality types (the impinger and the selector, similiar to the extrovert/introvert psychological concept) to allow for more complexity and scope.[8] Cumming emphasizes that the theory is not concerned with the special conditions of illness or poverty, but only with people of good health and adequate income. She argues that disengagement—initiated either by the individual or by others—eventually leads to a new equilibrium characterized by greater social distance and solidarity ties based on common values rather than on socioemotional roles and economic bonds.[8]

Cumming maintains that the shift away from achievement may cause a crisis in later years because of our social values. There is a need for new priorities. The ability to enjoy old age may depend on the ability and opportunity to use freedom. Disengagement is self-perpetuating; fewer contacts remain and more common values characterize the remaining contacts (churches, clubs, etc.). It is usually less disjunctive for women than for men. She suggests, finally, that disengagement is a return to individuation, which the child is encouraged to abandon—through socialization—to conform to social demands.[8]

This theory stirs the tempers of many gerontologists. They see it as an unjustifiable rationalization for social neglect and a misleading and harmful characterization of the elderly.

Others feel it may be helpful in understanding some of the behavior of the elderly. Arje believes the disengagement theory can be useful in tailoring rehabilitation techniques to old age.[9] She feels that disengagement may be a useful adjustment mechanism and, in some cases, is a guide to appropriate care. If withdrawal is normal, as the theory suggests, then the nurse must provide opportunities for socialization that offer pleasant, but not binding, interaction. More important, Arje finds this theory an aid in understanding those who are withdrawn people and in avoiding pushing or forcing interaction when it is not wanted.[9] The elderly person must be co-manager of his care, and a primary therapeutic goal is stimulating participation in self-care. She also emphasizes that, though withdrawal may be normal, increased activity may also be therapeutic in some cases.[9]

The disengagement theory is probably most helpful in those cases in which a nurse finds herself frustrated by a sense that her patient is indifferent to his care. This situation is sensitively described by Georges Simenon in *The Bells of Bicetre:*

> . . . it seems to us, I repeat, that you're not trying to get well, that you are being hostile to us . . . !
>
> Not hostile, indifferent. Even that wasn't the right word. He saw them different from the way they saw themselves. His problems were no longer the same as theirs. He had gone beyond them.[9]

Both the activity and disengagement theories have sharply limited applicability. People, as they grow old, are not always at the mercy of unvarying forces—either social or intrinsic—that they cannot control. They continue to make choices that are based on their experience and lifelong patterns, and "meat" for one is another man's "poison." Arje's applications[5] are crucial points to remember, but they do not depend on the disengagement theory for validity. They may be true *despite* the disengagement theory.

PRESENT SOCIOLOGIC THOUGHT

Sociologic study in the field of gerontology is fascinating and thought-provoking. Important points include the following:

1. Changes in time are both developmental and historical. Differences in age groups are due both to developmental stages (levels of activity, experience, etc.) and to historical circumstances. The historical experience of each generation has a lasting effect. For example, one generation of old people (75-year-olds) has continued to be conservative politically since they first voted in 1922. Many of them are foreign-born and uneducated. Some of the problems they encounter, such as

cultural loneliness, may not be prevalent in ensuing generations.

2. There are social as well as biological and historical time clocks. Age is a major dimension of social organization, both on the interpersonal and institutional level. Social age is related to rights and duties associated with seniority. Yet chronological age is an imperfect yardstick of social age. For one thing, we react to each other more in terms of status and position than in terms of actual years. One striking example is the difference between our treatment of a 60-year-old retired man and a 60-year-old nonretired man. Most workers must retire at 65, but Supreme Court justices may serve for life. In addition, life is often nonsynchronized; there is different timing in various areas of an individual's life. Many tensions arise from the social adherence to chronological age, in spite of other factors. Aging is most difficult in modern urban societies.

3. The aged are a quasi-minority group. There is discrimination in employment, aging is feared as a menace by the majority, and the aged often experience the feelings of self-consciousness, defensiveness, and self-hatred characteristic of minority groups. Those most prone to "minority" pigeonholing have the highest illness rate (though the relationship may not be causal).

Consider this man's comments:

> I am in my middle fifties and want to state that I regard myself a pretty good person and able to do a good day's work. . . . Some of the punishment I go through . . . regarding my age is sickly. Such remarks as "you old S.O.B., you're all washed up" at times make me want to do some harm . . . . One thing I notice when a younger person has authority over an older person: There seldom is any consideration.

4. Norms in old age become vague. There are very few specific norms for old age. Is this "normlessness" distressing or liberating?

5. There is a social breakdown syndrome. This syndrome is a theoretical model describing a social process of aging that leads to disease. Susceptibility or precondition to psychological breakdown, in combination with social labeling as deficient or

incompetent, leads to the induction of sickness or despondency, the atrophy of previous skills, a self-identification as sick or inadequate. This process is a vicious cycle, and may well operate in the aging of some people.

PSYCHOLOGICAL THOUGHT

Most general psychological thought applies to the elderly as well as to the young. Adaptive techniques such as denial, projection, or regression occur at all ages. This subject will be discussed more fully in Chapter 6.

One interesting clinical finding, specifically concerning old age, is that information-processing seems to slow with age, although intelligence functions as well or better. This may be due to a decrease in alpha rhythm frequency in the brain which is a physiological pacemaker influencing speed of response. Alpha frequency responds to conditioning (biofeedback); the old may be taught to speed up, and the young to slow down.[6]

CREATIVITY AND COMPETENCE

Perhaps nothing illustrates our common misconceptions about aging as clearly as the widely held views on reminiscing. Many people believe that reminiscence is a result of an old person's losing touch with memory of recent events. In contrast, reminiscence is properly seen as an important developmental task of old age.

This life-review process, in which memories of past experiences return with great clarity, is spontaneous, unselective, and probably universal. In old age, people remember sharply a whole train of long-ago events, especially conflicts and regrets that were never resolved. The life review is a natural healing process, in which a person's whole life is integrated. Goethe wrote: "He is the happiest man who can see the connection between the end and the beginning of his life."[1]

Life review is not always an easy process, especially because hardly anyone (besides grandchildren) is willing to listen to reminiscence. Remembering past conflicts so vividly often leads to anxiety, guilt, or depression; it may cause such pain that it leads to suicide.

On the other hand, when these conflicts are resolved inwardly, the life review leads to philosophical growth, often to wisdom and serenity and a lovely capacity to live in and enjoy the present. It also leads to creativity as an outlet for this newly won understanding. Many artists do their finest work in their later years, and many others discover creative abilities they did not know existed. According to Butler, "When a young man wants to write a novel, he resorts to autobiography. When an old man wants to write an autobiography, he may end up writing a novel."[10] What a treasure of knowledge we have in our old people, so much needed and so rarely tapped.

There are other qualities, common among older people, that deserve recognition and respect. Besides those already cited in this chapter and earlier, another instance is the "elder" function, in which older people may give advice to the young, which they feel their experience has verified.

Other common characteristics are a lively sense of the present (with less attention to future planning), and a joyful sense of curiosity and surprise which comes from living in the present. The elderly also often experience a sweet sense of fulfillment or consummation.

The freedom, the creativity, and the joys of old age should not be underplayed. They are a source of guidance for nurses and of satisfaction for the old. They are important to the older person's imaginative problem-solving ability and to his competence as an individual.

Bengston, a sociologist of the aged, has written that the task of the helping professions is to "enhance the *competence* of older individuals."[7] This goal is the key lesson of our understanding of the psychosociology of aging. Bengston lists three meanings of competence, three goals to pursue:

1. Competence means that the individual is enabled to perform his roles adequately. His independence and self-care are encouraged as much as possible.

2. Competence means that the individual is able to cope with his life, and to *do what he wishes to do.* The helping profession is responsible for helping people pursue their *own* goals.

(The Standards for Geriatric Nursing suggest this guideline: "The nurse finds out what the individual's lifestyle has been before she can determine that which is deviant."[11])

3. Competence is the feeling of doing well. The opportunity to take advantage of their experiences is often what gives older people a feeling of effectiveness.

In practical terms, this basic idea/orientation has specific implications. Nurses have the responsibility to recognize the continuity of the aging process at least as much as the losses involved. Strength must be acknowledged and experience respected.

We have the responsibility to recognize the creativity and freedom involved in the aging process and the growth and learning that are inherent in growing old.

It is our responsibility to agitate and advocate for needed social programs and for change in our cultural attitudes.

Social services do exist now, but many are inadequate. We have social security, health care subsidy, and some housing programs. A variety of retirement plans exist, but more are needed to provide adequate income. There is an urgent need for educational and recreational programs, and innovative ideas are now being started around the country. One example is day-care centers for the aged and infirm; another is special community college fees for the elderly. Social service programs, to be useful, ought to incorporate opportunities for growth, purposeful activity, self-reliance, and local responsibility.

A few institutions have highly successful, innovative programs. Moosehaven, in Florida, has a work program in which most of the residents participate; Cold Spring Institute, in New York, has creative, individualized programs planned by the residents for themselves.

Finally we need to give more responsibility to the aged themselves to make decisions about their own lives.

Old age depends on a balance of many factors. Loneliness may lead to malnutrition, which in turn may cloud reasoning ability. A grieving man may lose his job. Conversely, the freedom of old age, if given the opportunity, may lead to creative expression that enriches many lives. Care and attention may transform an isolated and lonely person into a satisfied and enjoyable friend.

To make a difference, we need to make commitments *as* human beings *to* human beings.

REFERENCES

[1]Butler, R. N. and Lewis, M. I.: *Aging and Mental Health.* St. Louis: C.V. Mosby Co., 1973, p. 106-107.

[2]Neugarten, B.L.: Grow old along with me! The best is yet to be. *Psychology Today*, 5 (No. 7): 46, December, 1971.

[3]Barron, M.L.: *The Aging American: An Introduction to Social Gerontology and Geriatrics.* New York: Thomas Y. Crowell Co., 1961, p. 69.

[4]Burnside, I.M.: *Psycho-Social Nursing of the Aged.* Workbook, Ethel Percy Andrus Gerontology Center, University of Southern California, Summer Institute for Study in Gerontology, 1974, p. 396.

[5]Kastenbaum, R.: Getting there ahead of time. *Psychology Today*, 5 (No. 7):53, December, 1971.

[6]Ethel Andrus Percy Gerontological Center: *Aging: Prospects and Issues.* University of Southern California, 1973, p. 77.

[7]Bengston, V.L: *The Social Psychology of Aging.* New York: Bobbs-Merril Co., Inc., 1973, p. 42.

[8]Cumming, E.: New thoughts on the theory of disengagement. *Int. Psychiatry* 6:1968. pp. 53-62.

[9]Arje, F.: Disengagement. A review of the theory and its implications for rehabilitative nursing with geriatric patients. *Nurs. Clin. N. America* 1:235–244, 1966.

[10]Butler, R.N.: The life review. *Psychology Today,* 5:7, 1971, p. 51.

[11]Standards for Geriatric Nursing. Executive Committee and the Standards Committee of the Division on Geriatric Nursing Practice. American Nursing Association, Kansas City, Mo. 1973.

SUGGESTED READING

Schaie, K.W., and Baltes, P.: Aging and IQ: The myth of the twilight years. *Psychology Today.* 7 (No. 10): 1974.

Chapter 3

The Physiology of Aging

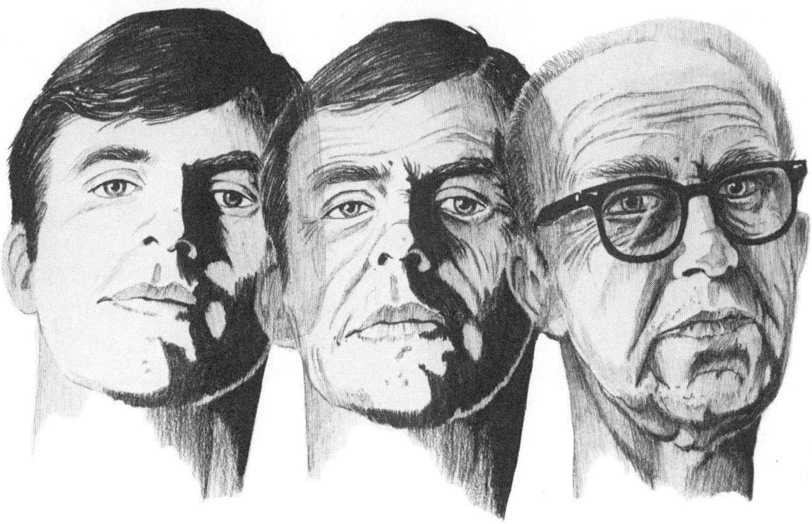

This chapter is devoted to the physiological process of aging: The changes— distinct from disease—that normally take place over time; the possible explanations for these changes; and the implications of these changes for nursing care. Although the focus is on physiology, it is important to bear in mind that human aging is comprehensible only when physical, psychological, and social forces are examined in interaction. There are physiological losses with time, but these are gradual, and there is usually more than enough capacity remaining for satisfying living. The degree to which the individual is able to use and nourish these capacities determines, in large measure, his total well-being.

Despite physical decline, most older people accommodate well to the aging process, coping more than adequately with daily challenges. People in the United States are living longer in better health. Moreover, many of the functional changes we normally associate with old age are not due to aging itself, but to disease or to disuse. Disease and disuse are often associated with psychosocial factors. The physical changes of aging may or may not lead to harmful consequences. These normal changes alone do not determine the degree of health in the aged person, though they do represent an overall decline in body function.

FUNCTIONAL CHANGES WITH AGE

Until 1951, very little was known about physical changes with age. Now extensive longitudinal studies have established five common characteristics of aging.[1]

1. Change is gradual.

Homeostasis is maintained fairly well in old age as long as disease is absent. The enormous reserve and redundancy of body tissue capacity preserve homeostasis despite some functional loss.

2. The more complex the function, the more decline is apparent.

For example, the decrease in the speed of nerve conduction is less than the decline in maximum breathing capacity. Nerve conduction is a simple physiological system, whereas breathing capacity involves the coordination of numerous systems.

3. Individual differences are significant.

There are great individual differences in the rates of aging and in the way people age. Furthermore, different tissue and organ systems age at different rates in the same person. Some physiological parameters change very little with age.

4. Vulnerability to disease increases.

People over 65 are twice as likely to be physically disabled; they are especially prone to cardiovascular disease, cancer, and cerebrovascular accidents.

5. Vulnerability to stress increases.

The single most critical age-related difference is the diminishing ability to respond to stress and return to the prestress level. In other words, there is a decline in homeostatic capacity. This is especially true for neuroendrocrine interaction; the degree of displacement is greater and the rate of recovery is slower. Stress may lead to disease more easily in old age, and there is ample evidence to suggest that disease may result from psychosocial stress as well as from physical stress.

These changes in the ability of the body to withstand stress are highly predictable. They seem to be independent of diet and other disease variables. The changes may be identified by the decrease of certain hormones in urine. One of the first measurable hormonal responses to stress is adrenocorticotropic hormone (ACTH), the tropic hormone of the anterior pituitary, which in turn stimulates the adrenal cortex to secrete the corticoids. Another measure of body response to stress is an initial rise in urine level of epinephrine and norepinephrine secreted by the adrenal medulla. These indicators make it possible to quantify the body's response to stress. Certain indicators of physical status, such as blood sugar, blood protein, pH, blood volume, heart rate, and blood pressure, may be relatively stable in aging, but under stress the capacity to maintain this stability declines.

There is more experimental evidence concerning the relationship of stress and aging. In studies of the mouse's capacity to withstand change in temperature, there is clear indication of decreased tolerance with age. Old people normally adjust relatively poorly to cold.

These are generalizations about the aging process. More specifically, there are common *observable* changes with age. The skin becomes thinner, less elastic, and more prone to wrinkles and pigmentation; the hair becomes thin and gray; the walk, slower; the frame shortens, settles, and becomes more brittle; the eyes often develop cataracts. What biological changes account for these oft-encountered conditions?

Aging occurs at different biologic levels. For example, the decline of muscle function is a sign of aging (the slower walk), as is a decreased capacity of individual muscle cells and the accumulation of certain substances within the cells. These functional changes will be examined by considering each of these levels separately, but briefly. All the changes are best understood within the context of the general concepts—that is, with an awareness of gradual change, individual differences, etc.

MOLECULAR AND CELLULAR CHANGES

Cells with regenerative capacity age in a distinctly different way from those which do not. Neurons and muscle and kidney cells do not reproduce. The loss of these cells over time may be responsible for functional changes in the brain, kidney, heart, and other muscle tissue. Redundancy in these organs compensates for some of this cellular loss.

Those cells which do regenerate—skin, liver, bone marrow, etc.—show a slower rate of repair with age. Chromosomal errors may accumulate as well, possibly resulting in faulty structural proteins or dysfunctional enzymes.

The intercellular connective tissue, which consists of collagen and elastin fibers, also changes with age, and some theorists postulate that these changes may interfere with intercellular exchanges and contribute directly to cardiovascular disease.

TISSUE CHANGES

Bone tissue often loses elasticity and mass, resulting in increased stress in weight-bearing areas. Muscle tissue characteristically decreases in both size and strength. Nervous and sensory tissue becomes less efficient in function.

SYSTEMIC CHANGES

Nervous System

Although simple neuronal function is relatively unimpaired, sensory sensitivity is often diminished. Tactile receptors are often less responsive, so pain or damage may not readily be perceived. The decline in taste and smell may affect nutrition. Taste buds for sweets often degenerate before those for other tastes. There is also a significant decline in space perception, and often in vision and audition. Perception of vibration decreases, as does responsiveness to temperature.

The most significant decrease is in the nervous system's integrative and coordinative capacity, often slowing speed of response. This may affect both physical and mental reaction time. It is the rate that is altered rather than the function itself.

Pulmonary System

There is a decrease in breathing efficiency, characterized by decreases in maximum breathing capacity, residual lung volume, vital capacity, and basal oxygen consumption, which leads to a lower overall metabolic rate. The result is fewer reserves for all body functions, since energy and nourishment require oxygen. Changes in the larynx may cause the voice to become weaker and higher pitched.

Digestive System

The amount of digestive enzymes, though still adequate, is reduced. Peristalsis is not as efficient, and constipation is often encountered. Such measures as small, frequent meals, and a diet including bran, prunes, and sufficient roughage frequently help to relieve these age-associated problems. Nutrition may be hindered by loss of teeth or by ill-fitting dentures, and anemia may result from a decreased absorption of iron.

Cardiovascular/Renal System

Usually a 55% decrease in blood plasma flow occurs between the ages of 30 and 80, and there are changes in the vascular walls. Peripheral resistance to blood flow may increase, elevating the blood pressure. Glomerular filtration, tubular excretion and stroke index often decline.

Endocrine System

Hormones (especially triiodothyronine and thyrotropin) decrease and those remaining do not elicit the same degree of response. Hormonal changes are of prime importance since they affect body metabolism. Some researchers believe that hormonal changes of the thymus gland are instrumental in the decreased ability of the aging body to generate antibodies necessary to fight infections.[2]

Sexual hormones also diminish over time in both sexes, although, of course, this change is drastic in female menopause. The gonadal decline may eventually produce a loss of male fertility, as well as in the female, but there is not necessarily a corresponding loss of libido in either sex.

Integumentary Changes

The loss of adipose tissue (the fatty connective tissue) and water undermine the skin foundation, causing sagging and wrinkles. Sebaceous glands are less active, resulting in dry or scaly skin. Lubricating lotions and less bathing and less need for soap may alleviate this condition. Areas of skin pigmentation are also common.

Summary

In summary, these physiological changes with age constitute a steady decline in functional capacity throughout the body. Perhaps the most significant alteration is the decline in the integrative function of the nervous system. However, adequate functional capacity remains intact, and the gradual pace of change encourages adaptation. Individual differences are marked, and the increased vulnerability to stress is considered of prime importance in the process of aging.

FROM THE INSIDE LOOKING OUT—A SUBJECTIVE PERSPECTIVE

All these observations of functional change come from a totally objective viewpoint. Yet what do we know of the internal experience of aging? To understand older persons, it behooves us to try to imagine how it feels to undergo these changes. How is physical aging perceived internally? What is the experience?

Of course, each individual response is different, but the reports of a few provide some illumination of subjective aging. Much of the following commentary has been drawn from *The Coming of Age,* Simone de Beauvoir's exhaustive work on aging.[1]

Old age is often difficult to recognize and accept because one is unlikely to consider one's self "old". Apparently a common experience is for the "self" to remain unchanged while the body ages. According to de Beauvoir, recognition of old age is largely forced upon the individual by the reactions of others. Repeatedly, people report being called "old" so regularly that they are compelled to come to terms with their own aging. At first, being called old is often a great shock; old age is regarded as something alien.

The body does send signals, but they are often ambiguous. Old age is often confused with disease; disease, with old age. Even when a condition is known to be a concomitant of age, such as rheumatism or arthritis, old age itself is not always fully recognized. The individual remains as he was always, with the rheumatism as something additional.

There have been a few studies devoted to how old people perceive their health, but the results are ambivalent. Some indicate that old people often consider their health to be poor; others give the opposite impression, that most old people consider themselves to be in good health even when seriously ill. Probably the most accurate opinion is one expressed by Professor A. Giusa at the Bucharest Geriatric Institute[3]: Old people often do not recognize disease as a condition distinct from age and adopt a passive attitude of renunciation toward their health.

There is some truth to the idea that "old age is somewhere between illness and health." Old age is, normally, a state of decline. It may be disconcerting and confusing, so the aging individual calls upon age to explain disease, and disease to explain aging.

Changes in physical appearance are the most certain evidence a person has of growing old. Others see him as old and he comes to see himself as old. We often hear stories of people meeting old acquaintances and being shocked by their appearance and then realizing, with grave apprehension, that their friend is also shocked. This change in aspect is difficult to accept, especially for women.

In time, the surprise seems to wear off. At 70, Jouhandeau wrote: "For half a century, I have persisted in being twenty years of age. The time has come to relinquish this unjust claim."[3] Yet for many, the genuine realization of old age is never made. In 1954, Tuckerman and Lorge interviewed over 1,000 Americans of various ages to find whether they felt young or old. Only a very small number of 60-year-olds felt old; after 80 years, 53% called themselves old, 36% middle-aged, and 11% young.[1] Often old age resembles a costume or mask which one is obliged to assume, although it does not project one's self.

These physiological changes with age often have an ambiguous meaning. The person inside the body evidently ages at a rate independent of his physiology. Perhaps we can say that individuals age at different rates: The organs age at varying rates within the body, but the person within that body ages at a still different rate. The older person is likely to have a very different self-image from the image seen by the observer. For this reason, an objective description of physiological aging without its subjective counterpart is an incomplete guide for nursing care.

THEORIES OF AGING

Understanding *what* happens in normal aging is very different from knowing *why* it happens. Man has been trying to discern the causes of aging for centuries, and much research is currently devoted to this question. It is possible that the numerous different theories, each focusing upon a different causative factor, are all correct. For example, it is valid to say that environmental conditions, such as a quiet, rural life, enhance longevity, and it is equally valid to suggest that genetic factors affect longevity. No one expects to find a single cause or explanation for old age.

The prominent theories of aging may be divided into two classes: external theories, which attribute aging to a variety of environmental factors; and internal theories, which attribute aging to physiological factors within the body. Several theories are reviewed in the Appendix at the end of this book.

Together the theories indicate that there is no single known biological mechanism that accounts for aging. The interplay of all these forces is a subject of research. One example of this interplay is the effect of menopause on other parts of the body. Menopause is an unusual example of an aging phenomenon consistently found in all populations, almost always occurring in human females between the ages of 40 and 50. Experiments have revealed that ovarian age is not responsible for menopause. Old ovaries placed in young mice continue to function normally. Signals from the pituitary or elsewhere in the body trigger menopause. Conversely, menopause causes aging symptoms elsewhere in the body. One common example is osteoporosis caused by lack of estrogen. It may be that there are aging "pacemakers" in the body—yet unknown—which govern the process of growing old.

Theoretical research on aging has practical implications for nursing care. An awareness of the scope and range of such studies is useful, for they accentuate the multiple factors involved in the aging process. The causes of aging are as varied and multidimensional as the functional changes. Those engaged in responsive health care can no longer simply categorize the aged patient as fulfilling general, nonindividualized expectations.

AGING AND DISEASE

This chapter would not be complete without a clarification of the relationship between aging and pathologic states or without mention of the inevitability of death.

Old age and disease are mutually related: age increases one's vulnerability to disease, and disease intensifies aging.

The incidence and severity of three major chronic diseases increase with advanced age. Cardiovascular disease, stroke, and cancer are the most widespread; other disorders occurring more often in old age include emphysema, rheumatism, arthritis, and broken bones. Most deaths caused by these diseases occur among the old, and these diseases most often appear in the last half to the last quarter of life. Age and disease are frequently coincident, yet no cause-and-effect relationship has been established between the two. Statistical evidence indicates an increased susceptibility to disease, yet the reasons for this relationship are really not known. One possible explanation is purely statistical: The longer one lives, the more challenges the body encounters. With increasing age, the ability to withstand these challenges decreases. Accidents increase with age; chronic diseases, symptomatic of the body's heightened vulnerability, also increase with age.

Others, notably Weg,[1] have tried to explain the high incidence of disease in terms of social and psychological factors. They emphasize the great amount of stress that characterizes the lives of most older citizens. Not only are older people often poor, lonely, and suffering from low self-esteem because of cultural neglect, they also often experience drastic life changes, such as loss of spouse, job, and home. There is a 75% correlation between the number of life change units on a "social readjustment rating scale" and the seriousness of illness. There is ample evidence to suggest that these changes may tax the coping capacities to the limit and result in a breakdown of adaptability and disease. In this way, it may be that the circumstances of old age are as much responsible for the high incidence of disease as the physiology of old age.

AGING AND DEATH

We do not die of old age, but of some challenge the body cannot resist. Since resistance declines while chances of challenge increase, it is inevitable that the risk of death increases sharply with age. Each individual ultimately encounters a challenge that his body is no longer equipped to resist. Cardiovascular disease is the most common cause of death in old age in the United States, accounting for 50% of mortality. The other common causes are essential hypertension and cancer; less widespread are respiratory disease and accidents. Interestingly, the three most common causes of death are often associated with the stress of civilized life.

The question of longevity is fraught with unknowns. It has been found that environmental factors influence the average life span of a population but not the maximum life span of an individual. Moreover, the major causes of death in any population may vary; in one, it is heart disease; in others, cancer or tuberculosis.

Leaf, among others, studied three isolated communities renowned for the longevity of their populations.[4] In Hunza, Pakistan, in the mountain village of Vilcabamba, Ecuador, and in the Abkhasian regions of the United Soviet Socialist Republic, people often survive in health and vigor for more than 100 years. There is a phenomenal lack of disease, and the aged are unusually active. These populations indicate that the maximum possibilities for a healthy long life are rarely fulfilled in most of the world, including the United States.

Scientists in both the Soviet Union and the United States have contrived similar lists of four predictors for increased longevity. They are (1) the maintenance of a positive life outlook and self-image, (2) a useful social role, (3) moderately good physical function, and (4) no smoking. How many of our old people can enjoy these conditions, particularly the first two?

THE IMPLICATIONS FOR NURSING CARE

An understanding of the physiology of aging has several concrete implications for health care. The most apparent lesson is that an open mind is essential: (1) individuals age at vastly different rates, (2) various organs also age at different rates, some—especially the more complex in function—being more vulnerable than others, (3) aging itself is not pathologic, and (4) outward signs associated with old age are often due to disease or disuse; therefore the nurse guards against prejudgment of geriatric patients. One crucial illustration of this is the fact that speed of response—both physical and mental—may be slowed although function is unimpaired. Older patients may adapt to physiological conditions that in younger people signify disease (such as high blood pressure), yet disease is just as "abnormal" for them as for any patient. One's own self-image of old age becomes operant here in making the distinctions between the norm and the pathologic state. Knowledge of common physiological changes may allow for more objective decisions.

The importance of stress and of the decline of capacity to respond to stress has significant implications. If a nurse is aware of sources of stress and can alleviate stressful conditions in some way, this is particularly therapeutic for an older patient. Conversely, we might expect unavoidable stress to affect the prognosis of an older patient more readily than a younger one. The decrease in capacity to regain homeostasis is often observable in older patients. Recognition that serious life changes can cause or exacerbate chronic disease may help to increase our sensitivity to the causes of disease in old age and suggest new therapeutic approaches.

Another important consequence of the physiology of aging is the necessity for special attention to nutrition and exercise. Changes in the digestive and pulmonary systems imply that the nutritional needs of the individual are increasingly difficult to meet, and a decline in the taste apparatus and in the condition of teeth may also hinder nutrition. Longevity studies show that exercise, activity, and a low-calorie diet may contribute significantly to health and longevity, and some theories also highlight the importance of nutrition in the aging process. A major responsibility appears to be providing sound nutrition and exercise whenever possible.

Sensory diminution also poses special nursing challenges. Older patients are often hard-of-hearing or suffer from impaired vision, and their care requires special approaches to counteract these conditions. The lack of tactile sensitivity indicates that pain may be experienced—and reported—less readily.

An awareness of the continuing sexuality of aging patients is also helpful in health care. Rather than dismissing the sexuality of aged people as inappropriate or absent, an acknowledgment of its rightful place in old age is beneficial.

Finally, an acknowledgment of the role of environment in the aging process is crucial. This fact has a two-fold meaning: In the first place, it is evident that living conditions and the patient's way of life are intimately linked to state of health. This information is applicable to health-care planning, and whenever appropriate, it should also be transmitted to the patient for cooperative planning. It means, too, that the hospital environment, including the positive attitudes of the nurse, is an essential part of clinical care. The nurse's sensitivity enhances the chances for optimal response.

REFERENCES

[1]Weg, R.B.: "Changing Physiology of Aging: Normal and Pathological." In Woodruff, D.S., and Birren, J.E.: Aging: *Scientific Perspectives and Social Issues.* New York: D. Von Nostrand Co., 1975, pp. 229-256.

[2]Walford, R.L.: "The Immunologic Theory of Aging." *Gerontologist* 4:195-197, 1964.

[3]Beauvoir, Simone de: *The Coming of Age.* New York: G.P. Putnam's Sons, 1972, pp. 283-340.

[4]Leaf, A.: "Getting Old." *Scientific American* 229:45-52, Sept., 1973.

SUGGESTED READING

Burnside, I.M.: *Psycho-Social Nursing Care of the Aged.* New York: McGraw-Hill, 1973.

Caldwell, E.: *Geriatric Nursing.* Albany, N.Y.: Delmar, 1972, pp. 27-33.

Curtis, H.J.: "A Composite Theory of Aging." *Gerontologist* 6:143-149, 1966.

Ethel Percy Andrus Gerontology Center: "Aging: Prospects and Issues." Monograph, Los Angeles: U. Southern California Press, 1973.

Spiegel, P.M.: "Theories of Aging." In Timaras, P.S. *Developmental Physiology and Aging.* New York: Macmillan, 1972, pp. 564-580.

"The Old in the Country of the Young." *Time* Aug. 8, 1970, pp. 49-54.

II

Caring for the Aged Ill

Chapter 4

Pathologic Conditions in Later Life

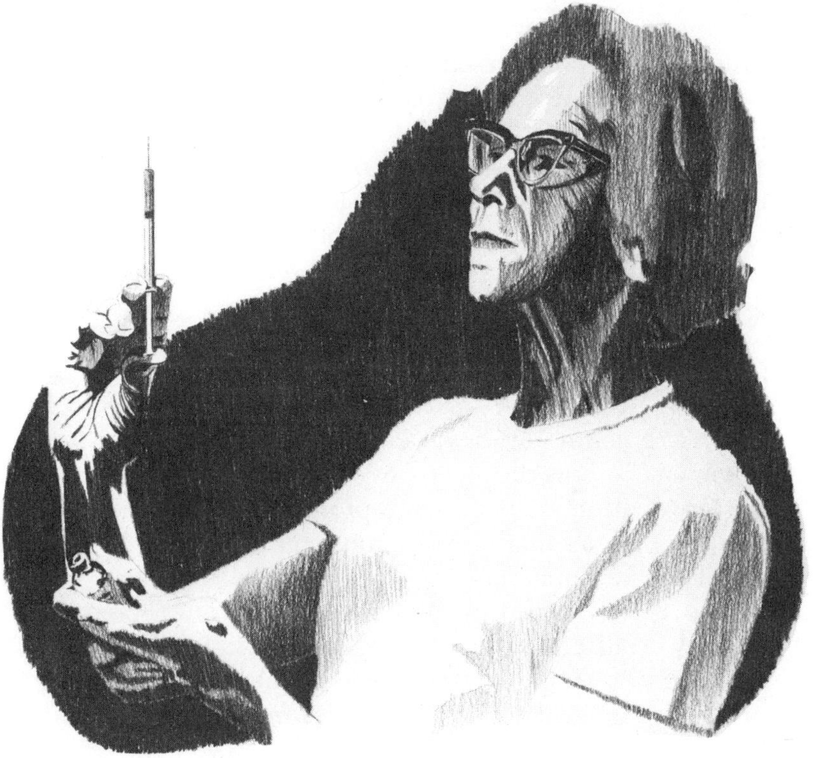

A familiarity with the normalities of aging, which we have emphasized thus far, provides a perspective from which to set realistic and individualized goals for nursing care. This chapter presents an overview of nursing practice for some common pathologies of old age, with a focus on appropriate interventions and frequently met problems in the care of older people, without a systemic review of geriatric pathophysiology. Particular attention is given to considerations for the use of drugs by the elderly.

Cancer and congestive heart failure are the two leading causes of death in persons over 65. Cerebrovascular accidents are the third. Advanced old age adds to the gravity of the prognosis in the seriously ill person, since the gradual degeneration of many bodily functions results in a diminished capacity to maintain and recover homeostasis. The care of the elderly person requires that clinical problems be assessed on a *daily* basis, in addition to consistent attention to the emotional needs of the patient.

CANCER

Cancer refers to a wide variety of conditions. There are more than 100 clinically distinct types of cancer now recognized, each having a unique set of symptoms and requiring specific therapy,[1] but all share three major characteristics: hyperplasia, anaplasia, and metastasis.

Hyperplasia is the uncontrolled proliferation of cells. The rate of proliferation is not higher, but rather the malignant cells fail to respond to the body's signals to halt division, thus producing a localized overaccumulation of tissue. The causes of hyperplasia are, as yet, unknown.

Anaplasia is a structural abnormality in which the cells resemble a primitive cell form, and in which mature cell function is absent or diminished, and the cell's spatial distribution may be jumbled.

Metastasis is the ability of a malignant cell to detach itself from a tumor mass and establish a new tumor in some other site in the body via the lymphatic or circulatory system. Metastatic tumors are more difficult to treat than nonmetastatic forms.

Although cancer is in many cases a terminal illness, it is not completely understood how cancer causes death. Malignancies seem to have a priority on nutrients within the body and result in generalized emaciation and illness. The direct cause of death is frequently infection; one study of 500 patients revealed that infection accounted for 36% of the mortalities. Hemorrhaging and blood clots accounted for another 18%.[1] More than half of all cancer deaths occur among persons over 65.

The prognosis for cancer varies greatly. At present, one-third of all cancer patients respond well to treatment. Early discovery and treatment is largely responsible for these successes. Many of the cancers common to the elderly are slow-growing and respond well to therapy when detected early. Cancer of the skin, often found in older persons, has an excellent cure rate (93% when treated promptly).[2] Preventive nursing care would therefore include inspection of all skin lesions in elderly patients, regular breast examination, routine Pap smears for those women who still have a uterus, and a chest x-ray yearly.

Probably the most important aspect of care the nurse can give the elderly cancer patient is emotional support. Almost everyone is frightened by the prospect of cancer, and patients often need to express their fear and their anger and frustration. Sensitive listening is desperately needed. This nursing function is critical for both the patient and the family and is often a bridge between the two.

Treatment for cancer currently involves three possible alternatives. Surgery, by conventional methods or through new techniques involving laser beams or cyroprobes is used to destroy or remove many forms of malignancies. Sometimes radical procedures such as mastectomies, laryngectomies, and colostomies are necessary. Patients undergoing such drastic surgery require special physical and psychological nursing support, and elderly patients may have an exceedingly difficult time adjusting to their new circumstances.

In any surgery involving a stoma, a nurse's patience and her unhurried, and encouraging attitude will help the patient learn the necessary skills for self-care. Emotionally, it may be easier for the postoperative patient to release his anger toward the nursing staff—or toward his family—than to direct it to the physician. Understanding and helping these patients express their feelings is a difficult nursing responsibility. Nurses need to come to terms with their own feelings about cancer and radical surgery to be able to accept and respond to the feelings of their patients.

Laryngectomized patients should be gradually encouraged to learn esophageal speech. In the interim, pencils and paper, a magic slate, and other means of communication should always be available. For some elderly persons, esophageal speech may be impossible, since it requires great concentration, control, and energy.

CARDIOVASCULAR DISEASE

Nurses today are independent decision-makers. They are assuming responsibilities once reserved for physicians. To assist the nurse in assessing the aged cardiac patient and in determining optimal care, Abbey has developed an organizing tool, FANCAP[3]: *F*luid, *A*ctivity, *N*utrition, *C*ommunication, *A*eration, *P*ain.

The following discussion focuses on the utilization of the FANCAP model with patients who are suffering from congestive heart failure or myocardial infarctions.

The common clinical symptoms of congestive heart failure are dyspnea, cough, rales, and fatigue. Mental confusion or restlessness, due to lack of circulating oxygen, is another manifestation of failure. Visible pulsations in the neck veins, ascites, dependent edema, or oliguria may also be present. The goals of care are to increase cardiac output and relieve the overburdened circulatory system. Basic therapy consists of rest and the use of diuretics and digitalis.

Myocardial infarction is the death of myocardial tissue due to lack of oxygen supply to heart muscle. Its major cause is atherosclerosis. Coronary atherosclerosis is a characteristic of normal aging, but it becomes abnormal when the collateral circulation can no longer compensate for the atherosclerosis. Myocardial infarction may occur with complete or partial coronary occlusion. Predisposing factors include age, diabetes, obesity, high serum cholesterol levels, and the use of tobacco. It may be precipitated by physical exertion, emotional strain, or severe blood loss.

In older patients, myocardial infarction commonly presents less pain than in younger persons, but occurs with more dyspnea and congestive heart failure. In later life, tolerance to myocardial infarction is lowered. Conditions indicating grave danger consist of severe shock, persistent dyspnea, severe cyanosis, persistent low blood pressure, acute left ventricular failure, rising fever, leukocytosis, arrhythmia, and congestive heart failure.[3]

The FANCAP model offers assessment guidelines and suggests appropriate interventions for both of these conditions. This model is particularly suitable for acute care, but may be modified for less severe conditions.

Fluid in Cardiovascular Disease

Edema. Cardiac disease often causes interstitial edema, which in turn may lead to pulmonary edema. Peripheral edema may cause skin breakdown and ulcers, since the fluid associated with edema contains not only water but toxic metabolic debris as well. The goal of care when edema occurs is to decrease capillary and pulmonary venous pressure.

Chair nursing is a useful intervention for edematous patients. Allowing the patient to sit up, with his feet on a chair for support, permits fluid to pool in the abdominal cavity and upper extremities. The patient's position must be changed frequently to avoid skin breakdown. Prolonged sitting in an upright position with legs dependent may result in peripheral edema; the nurse must take care to elevate the patient's legs slowly and moderately to prevent the rapid return of fluid to the heart and the possibility of right-sided congestive heart failure.

Skin and back care are very important for the aged patient. Back massage provides an opportunity to move and stimulate the patient. In edematous patients, the nurse must check for pressure points and reddened areas.

Intake. In the FANCAP model, fluid intake refers to all fluids, whether taken orally, parenterally, or in medications. Diuretics and digitalis, two components of the basic management of most cardiac conditions, are considered at this juncture.

It is often necessary to relieve the heart of added burden and to assist the kidneys' output through a diuretic regimen. This is especially true with older patients, since glomerular filtration rate and renal blood flow are reduced in the normal aging process. Water is the best—and the safest—diuretic. It should be given in small quantities at frequent intervals, and with an awareness that thirst is not always a reliable indicator of dehydration.

The use of diuretic drugs may induce a toxic reaction, producing a dangerous electrolyte imbalance, aggravating dehydration and elevating blood sugar and uric acid levels. Potassium depletion (hypokalemia), caused by stress, certain diuretics, vomiting, diarrhea, or malnutrition, may show itself through confusion or depression or through muscular weakness or irregular pulse. Hypokalemia also may enhance digitalis toxicity. The replacement of potassium is necessary, for if it isn't replaced, the situation may become life-threatening. Potassium chloride may be prescribed, or orange juice, bananas, or apricots may be added to the diet.

Digitalis therapy is often used in the management of cardiac disease because it increases cardiac output and thus slows heart rate. Its use must be carefully monitored. Older patients usually have increased sensitivity to digitalis and require smaller amounts. Any side effects, such as sinus bradycardia, arrhythmias, diarrhea, nausea, or visual changes, should indicate discontinuance. Digitalis may not be effective with elderly patients with badly damaged myocardium. It is useful to note that the apical pulse rate is the most reliable way to determine the need for digitalis.

Other drugs commonly prescribed for cardiac management include nitroglycerin, used in the treatment of angina. It is contraindicated for patients with glaucoma, as it increases intraocular pressure. Another is morphine sulfate, used for pain in myocardial infarctions and congestive heart failure. It may also alleviate the fear and restlessness associated with heart failure. Morphine has an antidiuretic action and depresses respiration. (It may alleviate Cheyne-Stokes respiration in congestive heart failure.) Demerol may be substituted for morphine when intense pain subsides.

Output. "Output," as used here, includes not only fluid output, but also information on vital signs and from laboratory studies. All fluid output, including emesis, should be recorded. Frequent emesis, perhaps drug-induced, may lead to dehydration and electrolyte imbalance. Urinary output is an important indicator of adequate circulatory function, and should be assessed not only for amount, but also for color, odor, and specific gravity. A reduction in amount may indicate renal complications or dehydration. Specific gravity provides information about the patient's level of hydration and kidney function as well. Daily weight is a good indicator of fluid balance, but it should be done at the same hour every day.

An increase in pulse rate may indicate hypoxia due to secretion accumulation in the lungs, infection, impending cardiac failure, or shock from reduced cardiac output or blood loss. Elevation of temperature is an early sign of infection, a serious complication in patients with cardiopulmonary abnormalities. An increase in temperature leads to an increased need for oxygen and imposes a greater burden on the heart and pulmonary system.

Activity in Cardiovascular Disease

Rest is a basic treatment for cardiac patients. It is, however, often ill-used. Excessive bedrest may lead to an increased venous return to the already overburdened heart, incontinence, constipation (and resultant heart strain), and infection. For patients with sufficient strength, chair nursing is the therapy of choice. Patients, especially those with congestive heart failure, are often more comfortable and relaxed, and so improve more rapidly, in a chair with arm supports. Chair nursing improves general circulation and decreases the risk of hypostatic pneumonia, thrombophlebitis, pulmonary embolism, and bed sores. Prolonged bed rest is often dispiriting as well; chair nursing is a morale-booster.

Early ambulation is now considered advantageous both physically and psychologically. It should be preceded by an assessment of cardiac rhythm and blood pressure. In general, though, the patient's activity level must be slower, it should be maintained.

> . . . The senior cardiac has more to fear from sedation, social segregation and senility than from cardiac disease . . . . Although the heart of the senior cardiac may be enlarged, its rhythm irregular and its reserve diminished, it is ordinarily capable of providing sufficient cardiac output for his needs.[4]

Specific nursing activity for cardiac abnormalities includes cardiac monitoring. It is important to combine a clinical assessment of the patient's condition with the use of a cardioscope to properly interpret the heart's output. Arrhythmias of particular concern are Stokes-Adams syndrome or complete heart block. A pacemaker is the most effective means of restoring cardiac function and is a lifesaver for many elderly patients.

No discussion of activity is complete without mention of mental activity. The patient needs mental stimulation and opportunities to relate to others and to express himself. Any deviations from the patient's normal behavior, such as confusion or restlessness, may signify biologic problems or drug toxicity.

Nutrition in Cardiovascular Disease

Nutrition, in the FANCAP model, involves both physical and spiritual needs. Physically, the patient's protein level must be maintained. It is important to provide an environment that enhances appetite (offer small servings if necessary) and assist in eating if needed. Low-salt diets may diminish appetite, and when coupled with diuretics, may cause hypokalemic alkalosis. Low-salt diets are often prescribed to regulate fluid balance, particularly during acute episodes and in severe cases of cardiovascular disease.

Glucose is the main source of cardiac energy. Elderly patients cannot tolerate even minor levels of hypoglycemia; in fact, high blood sugar levels are necessary. Diet should also include adequate iron to prevent anemia.

The spiritual needs of the patient, whether for religious counsel by clergy or for companionship, should be considered in addition to his dietary needs.

Communication in Cardiovascular Disease

Communication is the fourth parameter for assessment. It includes biologic communication, in the form of surgical or mechanical intervention when needed; environmental communication, in the form of structuring the patient's environment to protect him from infection and equipment malfunction, to provide a comfortable temperature, and to offer diversional activities and human-to-human communication. The aged patient needs personalized care, encouragement, and understanding.

Aeration in Cardiovascular Disease

Aeration refers to both oxygen therapy and the expression of feelings. Oxygen therapy is vital for acute stages of left ventricular failure, but oxygen may cause death in right-ventricular failure that is due to carbon dioxide narcosis.

The cardiac patient needs an opportunity to hyperventilate. It helps to allay his fears and reduces the risk of respiratory acidosis, while it helps the nurse to identify and alleviate sources of stress.

Pain in Cardiovascular Disease

Pain, either physical or psychological, is exhausting. All pain must be assessed in older patients to determine the appropriate intervention. The absence of pain when pain should be present is also significant, since it may indicate brain hypoxia.

The FANCAP model is useful with many other illnesses as well. Here, it has been applied to cardiac disease because cardiac abnormalities are so widespread among the aged.

CEREBROVASCULAR ACCIDENTS

Cerebrovascular accidents occur when blood circulation in the brain is impaired, causing the death of brain cells. Arteriosclerosis and hypertension contribute to strokes; heart disease, obesity, high blood cholesterol, and cigarette smoking are also predisposing factors. An attack may come without any warning, or it may be preceded by vague fatigue, headaches, or symptoms of "mini-stroke"—temporarily slurred speech, mild confusion, blurred vision, dizziness, or numbness of the hands.[5]

Nursing care for the stroke patient is chiefly concerned with rehabilitation. Immobility due to stroke may result in decubitus ulcers, contractures, and generalized weakness if preventive nursing care measures are not taken. All levels of disability—physical, intellectual, emotional and social—must be the concern of nursing services.

Five basic nursing services for stroke patients have been outlined.[6] It is emphasized that the staff must *first* develop an aggressive, positive attitude toward rehabilitation.[6] Restorative nursing focuses on encouraging activity, bladder and bowel training, nutrition, the prevention of contractures, and skin care.

Encouragement of Activity for the Stroke Patient

"Everyone on the nursing service must recognize that a stroke patient who is kept in bed will not recover."[6] Patients must be kept active, with gradual orientation to self-care. The encouragement of self-care must be done with sensitivity, to invite cooperation rather than resentment. Directions for activity should be stated simply and repeated patiently.

The goal of nursing care is to develop ambulation and encourage the activities of daily living as soon as possible, but rehabilitation is often a very frustrating experience for the patient. In giving instructions to stroke patients, it should be remembered that hemiplegia is often accompanied by emotional lability, confusion, and visual problems. Nevertheless, 85% of all hemiplegic patients can learn to walk and perform the activities of daily living.[5]

Bowel and Bladder Training for the Stroke Patient

An indwelling catheter is hazardous, even for patients with neurogenic urinary retention, because of the risk of infection.

It is possible temporarily to use menstrual pads with plastic pants for ambulatory women, and condom catheters for men. However, bladder and bowel retraining is an initial restorative step. A few measures achieve success in the great majority of patients. For bladder incontinence, a careful record of bladder incontinence will enable the staff to identify the times the patient usually voids and facilitate getting the patient to a commode. This enables the patient to function normally and maintain self-esteem. Adequate fluid intake should be given; an empty bladder is prone to infection and is more difficult to control. Bowel retraining is often aided by the addition of bran in morning breakfast cereals. It is helpful to set a daily schedule; normally, defecation occurs after a meal as a result of the stimulation of intestinal peristalsis by food intake. Bedside commodes with armrests and privacy are valuable pieces of equipment for patients who are unable to walk.

Nutrition for the Stroke Patient

Depression from immobility and illness often leads to a loss of appetite, and diet restrictions such as low sodium intake aggravate the situation. Meals are times of socialization to the average person. In a sense, there is a ritual associated with eating. Shared dining is extremely helpful to the improvement of appetite, socialization, and motivation toward self-care. If a dining room is inaccessible, eating in groups in the corridor is preferable to having the patient eat alone in his bed or in his room.

Prevention of Contractures for the Stroke Patient

It is the nursing staff's responsibility to get patients out of bed and to change their positions in bed frequently. It is important to position the patient with good body alignment immediately after the accident, during the period of flaccid paralysis. This reduces the degree of handicap when spasticity sets in. Passive range-of-motion exercise should be considered an adjunct to physical therapy, which nursing personnel can carry out to maintain functional mobility. One can take the initiative without a physician's order. In addition, patients may be encouraged to use the unaffected side to do passive range-of-motion exercises for themselves. To stimulate capillary circulation of the skin and to relieve body tension, massage and backrubs may be desirable.

In working with hemiplegic patients who had suffered strokes, pre-formed hard devices to position deformed hands or to prevent hand deformity may be more effective than the customary soft devices. One useful device consists of cones with a circumference of 6.5 inches on the wide end and approximately 4 inches on the narrow end, fashioned from firm cardboard. Kept in place with snug elastic, the cones exert a constant pressure over the entire flexor surface of the palms and fingers, decreasing flexor activity and increasing function potential of the hands. The cones are used all day and removed at night.[7]

Skin Care for Stroke Patients

Skin care is a cardinal nursing intervention, and crucial to the well-being of any immobilized patient. Procedures used to prevent decubuti are discussed later in this chapter.

Prevention of strokes—or of their recurrence—is a developing nursing function. Considerable research is being directed to identifying patients with "ministrokes," transient ischemic attacks (TIA). Eighty-five percent of TIA patients later have strokes, and the treatment of hypertension, hyperlipidemia, etc., is especially important for them. New diagnostic tools, monitoring equipment, and microsurgical techniques are being developed, and anticoagulant drugs are being used as an alternative to surgery for some TIA patients. In the meantime, nurses alert to TIA symptoms may reduce the severity, although not the incidence, of attacks.[8]

PARKINSON'S DISEASE

Parkinson's disease is a progressive illness affecting the motor nerves, which usually first manifests between the ages of 50 and

60 and runs a course of about 20 years. It afflicts 1.5 million people in the United States.[5] The chief symptoms are muscle rigidity, tremors, problems of the autonomic nervous system, a shuffling gait and a mask-like face. The loss of dexterity leads to difficulty in rising and initiating locomotion. Parkinsonian tremors are rhythmical and constant (usually five or six tremors per minute). Problems of the autonomic nervous system may lead to increased salivation, constipation, incontinence, decreased sexual function, and altered speech. These symptoms may cause the patient to withdraw. Depression, disorientation, hallucinations, and aggressive or suspicious behavior are not uncommon problems of patients with Parkinson's disease.

L-dopa is the drug of choice in the treatment of Parkinson's disease. The drug is effective in relieving some of the symptomatic tremors and rigidity of Parkinson's; in some cases, these symptoms disappear almost completely. In 75% of patients using L-dopa, according to one New York study,[9] symptoms improve by 50% or more. The use of L-dopa requires artistry because of its many side effects. Dosages must be individualized, and long-term patients may have great difficulty maintaining improvement. The drug does not cure the disease but only controls its symptoms. In some patients, L-dopa is not effective.[10]

Researchers are experimenting with other drugs (alphamethyldopa hydrazine and vitamin B_6) in conjunction with L-dopa. These agents seem to enhance or stabilize the effects of L-dopa. Again, the regimen must be highly individualized. Vitamin B_6 (pyridoxine) can counteract L-dopa. Patients should avoid legumes, powdered skim milk, sweet potatoes, avocado, wheat germ, and should eat oatmeal, pork, tuna, beef, liver, and dried fruits in moderation.

Side effects include gastrointestinal difficulties, muscle distortion, cardiac irregularity, and drastic involuntary movements. To control these complications, each patient must be assessed on a weekly basis to determine the ideal dosage. The side effects are usually most severe in elderly patients, and the greater the success in control of the symptoms, the greater likelihood there is that side effects will occur.

In Parkinson's, the goals of nursing care are to reduce muscle rigidity, to maintain a functional range of motion, and to maintain the use of upper and lower extremities. Active rehabilitation must be initiated at the outset of the disease to prevent contractures and resultant deformities.

The nursing-care plan requires a proper balance of rest and exercise. Fatigue aggravates parkinsonian symptoms and may contribute unnecessarily to frustration. On the other hand, adequate exercise is essential to preserving functional capacities and can reduce insomnia. The major portion of the patient's day is usually spent out of bed with occasional rest periods.

To assist walking, encourage the patient to touch the floor heel first, to keep knees straight and body erect, and to maintain a wide base of support. The nurse should be familiar with the instructions of the physical therapist to insure uniformity.[11]

Patients with Parkinson's disease are often intolerant to heat. They need light clothing and a cool room temperature. Nourishment is very important to reduce progression of the disease, but eating may be difficult. For reasons of socialization, the patient should be encouraged to eat in company and to feed himself for as long as possible. He should be given foods that do not spill. Foods that may lead to constipation must be avoided. (In later stages of Parkinson's, self-feeding is not possible. Careful assistance in feeding is necessary, as the patient may have difficulty chewing and swallowing.)

Maintaining independence as long as possible will provide the patient with a therapeutic range of activity. *Every activity helps prevent further rigidity.* If handwriting becomes impossible, typewriting is often feasible and is good exercise. Group therapy is often helpful, and speech therapy exercises should be encouraged to maintain speech facility.

Learning to cope with Parkinson's disease is a long and trying process. The patient will experience periods of frustration and needs generous doses of encouragement, reassurance, and understanding. Stress and anxiety aggravate the symptoms and should be reduced whenever possible. Parkinson's may cause emotional instability, and crying should be accepted behavior. Perhaps most important, Parkinson's disease does *not* impair mental capacity although it causes speech difficulties and a mask-like expression. The patient craves intellectual stimulation and needs social acceptance. Small acts, such as a touch, a smile, and relaxed conversation, are important.

OSTEOARTHRITIS AND RHEUMATOID ARTHRITIS

A widespread degenerative joint disease, osteoarthritis afflicts between 70 and 88% of the population over 65.[12] The disease is caused by the degeneration of cartilage in the joints, gradually making movement of the joint difficult and painful. It affects the joints of the hips, knees, the vertebrae, or at times the hands, feet, and shoulders. Although occasionally found in a young patient, osteoarthritis is predominantly a disease of the middle and late years. Joints that have been damaged or strained are *especially* susceptible. Osteoarthritis is probably due to the wear and tear on the joints from long use; it is not systemic.

Osteoarthritis usually remains rather mild when small joints are involved, but may cause intense pain and severe limitation of motion in such joints as the hip. For these severe cases, total hip replacement surgery is sometimes recommended. Commonly, treatment of less severe osteoarthritis relies on analgesics such as aspirin, occasional corticosteroids, and the relief of stress on the affected joints by rest. Loss of weight is often indicated to relieve stress, and physical therapy, such as range-of-motion exercises, may be helpful.

Rheumatoid arthritis is a far more debilitating disease. It is not a disease of the aged, but more often begins in young adulthood. Yet many older patients have serious problems with mobility as a result of repeated bouts of rheumatoid arthritis. Nursing care should emphasize encouraging mobility and inventive solutions to daily self-care problems.

DIABETES MELLITUS

Diabetes in adults appears most often in the seventh decade of life. The discovery that one has diabetes can be an emotionally painful and alarming experience, and a thorough explanation of the disease and its control is essential. The patient must understand his dietary requirements, how to administer insulin or oral hypoglycemics if necessary, how to test urine, and how to recognize symptoms that require immediate medical attention.

Sugar in the urine means that there has been an insufficient supply of usable insulin to metabolize all the sugar; ketone bodies, the by-product of fat metabolism, indicate that glucose is not being metabolized and that the body is drawing on its supply of fat to provide energy.

The main goal of nursing is to help the patient understand his disease, control his therapy and adapt his life style. In older people, instructions should be given slowly because the patient's speed of comprehension may be diminished. Pamphlets from the American Diabetic Association, books, and group meetings may be helpful.

The management of diabetes in the elderly may not require insulin. Careful diet and/or oral hypoglycemic agents often suffice. Diet is especially important in the care of older people. Obesity is directly related to diabetes in older adults. In the elderly, borderline diabetes or glucose intolerance is not uncommon and should be fully explored.

Changing a diet of long standing may require considerable nursing support. A sense of humor can really help both nurse and patient:

> Julia developed diabetes while she was living at a convalescent hospital. At first, she required insulin, but eventually she was able to control her condition with a careful diet. Julia was exceedingly fond of cough drops, and her doctor decided she might have some if the nurses would bring her three at a time a few times a day. A lady of great spirit, she was quite irate about this dole method, but she went along with it to get her cough drops.
>
> One evening, a nurse looked up from her chart work to see Julia sighting down the "barrels" of her pointed fingers.
>
> "This is the geriatric bandit," she exclaimed. "Give me my pellets!"

The most common symptoms of the onset of diabetes are *polyphagia,* without a corresponding weight gain; *polydipsia,* which might be recognized by such statements as "I seem to be thirsty all the time" "I seem to be always drinking so much water"; and *polyuria,* which does not necessarily relate to the increased fluid intake. Other signs of the onset of diabetes may include easy fatigability, slow healing of cuts, frequent infections, itching, burning on urination, due to the irritation caused by unmetabolized glucose in the urine, and visual changes. Any of these problems may occur singly or together.

Hypoglycemia is infrequent in the elderly, but it may occur swiftly and be fatal. It is the result of too much insulin in the body, in relation to the amount of glucose available, and can precipitate heart attacks or strokes. Classic symptoms are usually not experienced by older patients. They instead may exhibit bizarre or unusual behavior or become unconscious without warning. At night they may experience nightmares or restlessness. Orange juice or other sugar should be given immediately, or intravenous glucose if the patient is unconscious.

Diabetic coma (ketoacidosis) occurs when there is an inadequate amount of insulin to metabolize the amount of glucose in the body. It may be caused by the patient's failure to take routine insulin, by overeating, or by infection, which creates a greater energy demand on the body. Certain drugs increase the danger of ketoacidosis; these are cortisone, its derivatives, and some diuretics. Symptoms of diabetic coma are deep rapid respiration, a flushed face, and red, dry skin, a state of confusion and stupor resembling drunkeness, and sweet fruity breath (acetone). It is not uncommon for comas gradually to develop, with symptoms of headaches, drowsiness, and confusion.

In the aged, diabetes may contribute to other pathologic conditions. It apparently encourages the deterioration of the cardiovascular system. Neuritis and neuropathy, including mental impairment, are not uncommon. Diabetes predisposes the patient to vascular disease, especially in the eyes, kidneys, and lower extremities. The diabetic person needs adequate diet and exercise, sound weight control and regular preventive care. Forethought should be given so that these basic requirements are not inhibited by the economic and social circumstances of old age.

MULTIPLE PATHOLOGIC CONDITIONS

In the aged, multiple illnesses frequently present special problems for nursing care. A patient may have both rheumatoid arthritis and Parkinson's disease. In this case, since both conditions benefit from activity, nursing intervention should revolve around self-care and mobility. On the other hand, a patient may suffer from congestive heart failure and an arthritic condition. Both these conditions require rest, but stiffness from arthritis may ensue from inactivity. This kind of contradictory situation calls for imaginative solutions that include the patient in the problem-solving process. Chair nursing may be beneficial in this instance. In most cases of multiple illnesses, the key to nursing care is thoughtful, optimistic experimentation and patient cooperation, focused on assisting the patient to a realistic optimal level of functioning.

DECUBITAL ULCERS

Many chronic conditions cause immobility, yet they need not cause decubiti. Skin care is exclusively a nursing responsibility, and successful action requires staff coordination and motivation. The entire staff needs information and a standardized treatment plan to avoid decubiti. Everyone has to be aware of the need for care in removing bedpans, ensuring that the patient is free from residue body waste, and for quickly changing sheets and dressings that are wet or soiled.[13]

Foam protectors for heels and elbows have been used to prevent decubiti.[14] Heavy-duty foam, 6 or 7 inches thick, cut to fit the contour of the body part and covered with muslin, are helpful for unresponsive or paralyzed patients. Sheepskin protectors and foam pads may also help.

Basic prevention of decubiti involves two steps: The first is insuring that the patient receives adequate nutrition, since emaciation makes decubiti unavoidable; the second is the frequent changing of the patient's position, and checking and caring for pressure points and reddened areas regularly.

DRUGS AND THE AGED

Older people often use drugs routinely and for long periods in the treatment of chronic illnesses. Ten percent of the population, the elderly use 25% of all drugs.[15] No drug is devoid of toxicity, and the elderly have a significantly lower tolerance to drugs. Normal physiological changes in old age influence the absorption, distribution, metabolism, and elimination of drugs, often resulting in a greater concentration of the drug at the site of its activity and longer effects. Dosage tolerance is lower especially with drugs whose elimination depends on kidney function. This leads, in turn, to a greater likelihood of adverse reaction. The interaction of multiple systems at peak tolerance in old age makes the elderly especially vulnerable to drug toxicity.

Therefore, it is not surprising that adverse reactions to drugs pose a serious health hazard to the aged population. Proportionally more older people are admitted to hospitals as a result of adverse drug reaction, and in the hospital, more elderly patients have drug reactions. Many adverse drug reactions may go unrecognized. Mental disturbances are often the first sign of toxicity. A nonspecific failure to thrive (*i.e.*, deteriorating physical condition and social competence) may also result from adverse drug reaction. Multiple diseases, with multiple drug therapies, compound the problem.

Research has shown that errors of commission or omission in the self-administration of drugs is not uncommon, especially with elderly patients using long-term multiple drugs. Erratic dosage and overdoses may manifest first in mental changes. One study found 59% of an elderly, chronically ill outpatient population made errors of this kind.[15] It is clear that nurses should take great care that instructions concerning medications are understood by the patient.

The occurrence of medication errors is not limited to self-care. One medication error has been reported to have taken place for every six doses administered in an acute hospital setting.[11] Limited information about errors in nursing homes suggests a 14–32% error occurrence in skilled nursing facilities.[15]

Acute brain syndrome, reversible if treated, is frequently related to drug use. The elderly are especially vulnerable to an adverse reaction to psychotropic drugs (atropine-like), anticholinergics, used for Parkinson's disease and peptic ulcers, antidepressants, and sleep and cold preparations.

Central nervous system depressants warrant special attention. They may cause oversedation in elderly patients and may precipitate pneumonia.

Digitalis toxicity, mentioned earlier in this chapter, is one of the most common and serious drug-induced diseases. Adverse reactions also occur frequently with diuretics and oral hypoglycemics. All drugs should be monitored with care, and any erratic mental behavior should alert the nurse to possible adverse reactions.

CONCLUSION

Illness in older patients is often complicated by the patient's fear of death or of long-term disability. An old person is usually acutely aware of his body's increased vulnerability, and it is understandable that he may react to disease with deep anxiety. Such worry and fear, we know, adds an additional stress to the aged patient's already overburdened system. Nurses, through personalized holistic care, can comfort their patients and share with them a sense of calmness and companionship.

REFERENCES

[1]"What is Cancer." *Science* 183: 1069, 1974.

[2]Caldwell, E., and Hegner, R.: *Geriatric Nursing.* Albany, N.Y.: Delmar, 1972.

[3]Roberts, S.L.: "Cardiopulmonary Abnormalities in Aging." In *Nursing and the Aged.* Edited by I.M. Burnside. New York: McGraw-Hill, 1976.

[4]Harris, R.: "Special Features of Heart Disease in the Elderly Patient." In *Working with Aged People.* U.S. Dept. Health, Education and Welfare, Vol. 4, 1971.

[5]Birchenall, J., and Streight, M.E.: *Care of the Older Adult.* Philadelphia: J.B. Lippincott Co., 1973.

[6]Mead, S.: "Stroke Rehabilitation." In *Stroke and Its Rehabilitation.* Continuing education monographs, San Francisco: 1975, p. 42.

[7]Dayhoff, N.: "Soft or Hard Devices to Position Hands?" *Am. J. Nurs.* 5: 86-88, 1975.

[8]Burnside, I.M.: *Nursing and the Aged.* New York: McGraw-Hill, 1976.

[9]"Concerted Scientific Effort Toward Better Use of L-Dopa." *Medical World News,* March 3, 1972.

[10]"The Story of L-Dopa from Observation." National Parkinson Foundation, Miami, Fla.

[11]"Exercises for the Parkinson Patient." Parkinson's Disease Foundation, New York, N.Y.

[12]Blau, S.P., and Schultz, D.: *Arthritis.* Garden City, N.Y.: Doubleday, 1974.

[13]Fleming, A.S.: "Motivating a Staff Plagued by Failures." *Nursing '75.* 5: 86-88, 1975.

[14]Yentzer, M.: "Conquering those Obstinate Decubiti." *Nursing '75,* 5: 1975.

[15]Kayne, R.C.: "Drugs and the Aged." In *Nursing and the Aged.* Edited by I.M. Burnside. New York: McGraw-Hill, 1976.

SUGGESTED READING

Hodkinson, M.A.: "Some Clinical Problems of Geriatric Nursing." *Nurs. Clin. Am.* 3: 657, 1968.

Marino, E. B.: "Vinnie was Dying." *Nursing '74,* 4:46, 1974.

Ritchie, M.: "Heart Failure—the Geriatric Patient." *Nurs. Clin. Am.* 3:663, 1968.

"Symposium on Putting Geriatric Nursing Standards into Practice." *Nurs. Clin. Am.* 7:1972.

Wheeler, D.V.: *Aggressive Nursing Management of Acute Myocardial Infarction,* Philadelphia: Charles Press, 1968.

Chapter 5

Problems in Communication

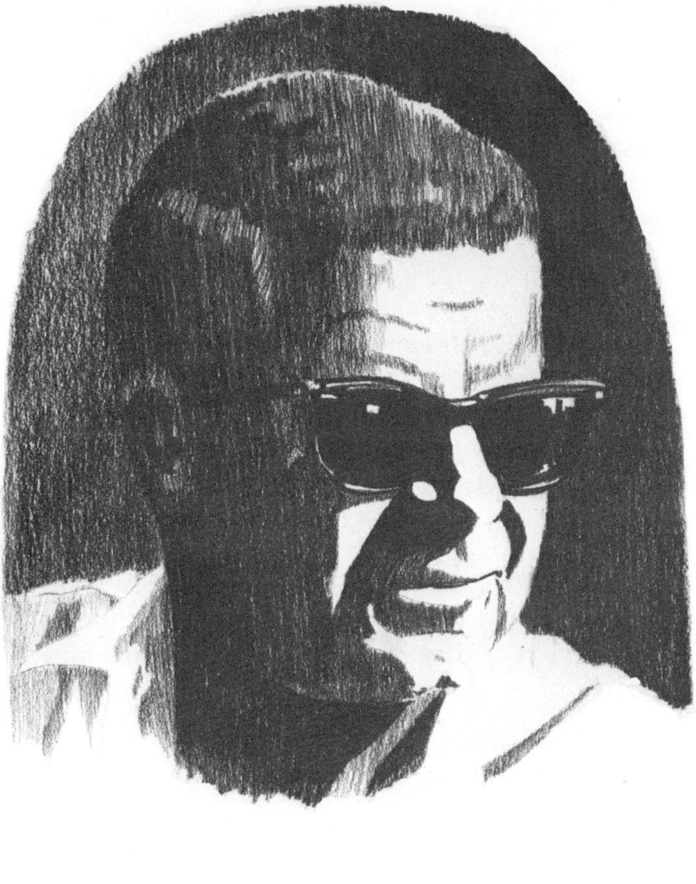

There is no therapeutic relationship without communication. Care of the elderly is often complicated by communication disorders, in the forms of blindness, deafness, or aphasia. Communication is necessary to personalized care-giving, and it is essential to assist those afflicted with one or more of these disabilities to lead full, satisfying lives.

Genuine communication with elderly patients who have *no* such disability is too often neglected. It is, of course, much more difficult to establish patterns of communication with those who do. Without encouragement to communicate, these disabled and aged individuals are left isolated, lonely and frightened. Helping them to communicate is one of the most salutary aspects of geriatric nursing.

BLINDNESS

Almost half of all known cases of blindness occur in people over age 65.[1] Vision is constantly used in communication, to record facial expressions, nonverbal cues, and to identify the speaker. Loss of vision affects communication with others as well as creating more obvious problems with mobility and self-care. Blindness decreases social contact by lessening stimuli from books, newspapers, television, and card games, all of which, in standard form, require sight.

It is helpful to keep in mind two facts about visual impairment. First, persons who are legally blind may have a small degree of residual vision. This means that you, as a care-giver, must frequently make use of whatever vision remains to help the person adjust to his environment or to teach a particular skill. Therefore, it is important to assess the extent of a person's residual vision as soon as possible and to encourage its use. Many elderly people are reluctant to use their eyes, fearing to lose what remains of their vision. Sincere reassurance by those whom they trust may allay this fear.

The second fact is that the blind person's vision may fluctuate, being better one day than the next, or better in daylight than at night. Learning to function with fluctuating vision is more difficult than adjusting to a consistent visual impairment. Again it is important to assess not only the amount of residual vision the patient possesses, but whether fluctuation is present.

Causes of Blindness in Old Age

There are four major causes of blindness common to the elderly; glaucoma, senile cataracts, optic macular diseases, and diabetic retinopathy. Nearly all older people need glasses as the elasticity of the lens of the eye decreases, beginning in middle age. This causes a form of farsightedness known as presbyopia. Despite presbyopia, 80% of the elderly have reasonably good vision. The aged usually fear and dread the loss of vision; many believe blindness to be much more widespread in old age than it actually is.

Yearly examinations are recommended for older people, and immediate care should be sought when signs of trouble occur. These are early symptoms:

1. Redness, irritation, or excessive watering
2. Decrease in tearing, or dry eyes
3. Frequent headaches
4. Visual disturbances, such as spots, halos, or blurs
5. Loss of peripheral vision

Observation of the elderly's behavior may be the first clue to eye problems. For example, decreased peripheral vision may be manifested by their bumping into things or walking close to walls to provide a guide for the route. Some changes are so gradual that the person afflicted is unaware of the change; others are rapid and evoke a comment of alarm.

Glaucoma. Glaucoma is a condition in which the fluid pressure in the eye is too high. It occurs in 2–4% of the adult population, usually in the elderly. There may be a familial tendency toward glaucoma. Symptoms may include headaches on one side of the head, blurred vision, and rainbow halos around light bulbs. Peripheral vision is lost first, and then central vision is affected.

In its acute form, glaucoma may cause acute eye pain, headache, and nausea. Eighty to ninety percent of glaucoma cases are chronic and painless, and the loss of vision is gradual. It may go long unnoticed. Bending, lifting, use of tight-fitting clothes, and emotional tension all tend to elevate intraocular pressure and should be avoided by persons who are afflicted with glaucoma.

Senile cataracts. Senile cataracts are usually found in people over 70. The loss of vision is due to a gradual increase in the opacity of the lens. Causes include the degenerative processes of age, disease, drugs, and irradiation, among others. Sometimes double vision or color blindness is symptomatic of cataracts. Treatment of cataracts by their surgical removal and the wearing of specific prescription glasses has resulted in about a 95% success rate.

Care of a patient about to undergo cataract surgery includes preparation for temporary blindness after the operation. It is important to acquaint the patient well with his room and with hospital services beforehand. The postoperative adjustment period is quite long, usually 6 weeks to 3 months, and recovery depends in large part on the patient's morale. The nurse's positive and supportive attitude is important.

Macular diseases. Macular diseases include such conditions as arteriosclerosis, hypertension, nephritis, some parasitic diseases, and some central nervous system disorders. The macula is a small part of the retina responsible for the clearest central vision; it is more vulnerable in the aging person.

Diabetic retinopathy. Diabetic retinopathy can cause hemorrhaging of the capillaries in the eye. Not all persons with diabetes suffer from this incapacitating disorder, but frequent eye checkups are important for early detection.

Personal Contact

The American Foundation for the Blind has published some guidelines for offering help to the aging blind person.[1] They point out that an aged individual's reaction to blindness depends on his personality, his life style and general outlook, his ability to purchase services, and how many of the losses of old age he has already experienced.

1. If blindness comes suddenly, a period of depression and withdrawal is a *normal preliminary* to emotional recovery. The patient needs support, understanding and gradual encouragement toward rehabilitation.

> The difference between whether he spends his life sitting in boredom or whether he is able to get around and do the things that interest him may depend on how well he learns the techniques that have been developed to help blind people achieve orientation, mobility, and skills for daily living. How well he learns these techniques, or how interested he is in learning them, depends a good deal upon his attitude towards his visual handicap and the encouragement others give him.[1]

The attitudes of those working with the patient will have a strong influence on his own attitudes.

2. It is important to know the blind person as an individual. Stereotypes—either of age or of blindness— should be avoided.
3. The aging blind person must learn to rely on the remaining senses. This is no automatic skill, but one slowly learned, because vision is not independent of the other senses. For this reason, hearing should be evaluated and any residual vision should be protected.
4. The patient needs love, friendship, and acceptance. The older person may take longer than a younger person to accept help from someone he does not know. His own opinions of his needs should be respected.
5. The blind person must make decisions about how to conduct his life, degrees of dependency, and how to ask for help. It is best to let him decide, to foster self-reliance as much as possible. Avoid rigidity in your relationship with him, and in solutions to problems.

The American Foundation for the Blind also has concrete suggestions about day-to-day contact with the elderly. Caregivers should address the blind person by name to let him know when he is being spoken to and when he is being left. He should be told who is speaking, and forewarned of activities or hospital procedures such as injections. There is no need to speak loudly, or to use his companion as a "translator."

When teaching a particular skill, make your directions simple and consistent. Whenever possible, use touch to replace sight. Allow the blind person time to learn.

Techniques for teaching basic skills are explained very clearly in the manual, *An Introduction to Working With the Aging Person Who is Visually Handicapped.* This book, by the American Foundation for the Blind, is very useful for teaching blind people walking techniques, eating, handling money, shaving and brushing the teeth, sewing, selecting clothes, and much more. It describes in detail how to teach people to feed themselves, to smoke independently, and to sign their signatures.

For example, an easy way to describe the placement of food on a plate is the clock method—peas at 6 o'clock, potatoes at 2 o'clock, bread is outside at 9 o'clock, etc.

In room familiarization, the guide uses the door as a reference point in giving right or left directions and in relation to other objects in the room. The guide describes the shape of the room, the location of windows and other doors, the general contents, and perhaps the colors and styles. The location of radiators, ashtrays, and the thermostat is also indicated. The blind person is guided slowly around the room and allowed to touch edges and furniture. The blind person will feel more at ease by learning to move freely about the room.

Low vision aids of many kinds are available for the use of the legally blind. These include magnifying glasses, telescopic devices, and closed-circuit television systems to enlarge images. Proper lighting appliances often aid partial vision. Books and telephone dials are available in large print, and, of course, there is a great deal of Braille information and reading material available.

Devices such as Brailled watches and clocks, raised numbers for doors at eye level, syringes for diabetics, signature guides, and a wide variety of puzzles, playing cards, and games such as Scrabble, bingo, chess, and checkers (for sighted and sightless) are available from the American Foundation for the Blind.

The elderly blind often require special help with transportation and home health care. Local health and welfare offices or the United Fund will be of service here, as well as special agencies for the blind listed in American Foundation for the Blind publications.

DEAFNESS

Significant hearing loss occurs in 30% of all older people; men more often than women are affected.

Deafness has been called "potentially the most problematic of the perceptual impairments."[2] Deafness is often found to be a cause of suspiciousness, even of paranoia. It may lead to extreme social isolation with severe emotional consequences.

Presbycusis is the progressive loss of hearing due to age. It has been correlated with environmental noise; city life contributes to earlier hearing loss. In the absence of a noisy environment, presbycusis does not occur. In a study of the Mabaans of Sudan, a very isolated, quiet tribe who do not even use drums, very little hearing loss was found in the elderly.[2]

Hearing loss is often so gradual that it is long unnoticed. Older people may deny that they have difficulty hearing, or they may accept deafness as an inevitable part of aging. Since causes for diminished hearing include infections, diabetes, drugs, or impacted wax in the ears, referral to an otologist is advisable. In some cases, hearing aids are very useful, but when there is nerve degeneration, hearing aids do not help. Interestingly, Nei Ching Acupuncture Center in Washington, D.C. reports significant success with acupuncture as a treatment for nerve deafness.

Personal Contact

Because the elderly often lose hearing ability gradually, it is a good idea to check hearing whenever a person becomes more difficult to talk to, responds inappropriately, plays the radio loudly, etc. *Early diagnosis may be important to treatment.*

High-frequency sounds are lost before low-frequency sounds, and consonants are high-frequency sounds. Without the consonants, language becomes disjointed, and much misunderstanding ensues. Imagine any simple sentence without clear consonants—hOw ArE yOU tOdAy—and it becomes clear why communication can become so difficult.

When talking to a person who is deaf or hard-of-hearing, always touch him before speaking to gain attention. Enunciate carefully and slowly and be sure to stand so that your face is unobscured. Lip-reading is very helpful to some people, but don't rely on it, especially with people who may have poor vision as well. Listen carefully and get used to the individual's particular speech pattern, as hearing loss affects the ability to speak clearly. Do not pretend to understand if you don't. Discover which ear has the better hearing and speak close to it. There is no need to shout or to speak exceptionally loud. This only creates high-frequency sounds, the sounds that are the first lost in hearing impairment. It is useful for nurses to familiarize themselves with hearing aids worn by their patients—understanding how they work, checking the batteries often, and checking the patency of the ear mold on those that fit into the ear canal. All too frequently wax forms a plug, decreasing the aid's effectiveness.

Hearing is so crucial to mental health in old age that this factor deserves special emphasis. Deafness causes even greater social isolation than blindness, since it hinders verbal communication, and it is generally met with less social sympathy. The deaf are often excluded from activities; deafness may even be confused with senility. Thus, the emotional impact of deafness can be severe. Seventy percent of the aged who are admitted to psychiatric facilities have hearing loss.[3] Deafness is related to depression in older men, according to National Institute of Mental Health studies.[2] It is also commonly a physical factor in paranoid schizophrenia in elderly patients. It is related to slower reaction time.

People with hearing loss are prime victims of projection, an adaptive technique in which feelings are projected outward onto someone or something else. Projection signifies anxiety, and can reach paranoiac proportions unless the inner stress is somehow reduced. Another adaptive behavior frequently observed in the elderly deaf is selective reception, a process of excluding some sounds or undesirable information while receiving others.

It is difficult—sometimes annoying—to try to converse with people who have impaired hearing. Yet it is important to try to counteract, to some degree, the isolation of deafness.

Hearing aids of many kinds are now available, but a comprehensive evaluation of each person's hearing is a prerequisite to finding the correct prosthetic help. Other available technologic aids are amplifiers for phones (usually available at little charge from the phone company), vibrating pillow alarm clocks, teletype communication systems attached to phone lines, and other vibrator alerting devices. These may be invaluable for particular home health care problems.

APHASIA

Each individual's aphasia is unique. There are, however, three general categories which are useful for patient evaluation.

1. *Expressive aphasia* prohibits speaking or reading aloud, but patients can hear and understand language, and may be able to say yes or no.
2. *Receptive aphasia* is more complicated—it includes loss of comprehension of the spoken or written language, and the patient may speak volubly but misuse words. Rehabilitation is complicated by the fact that this kind of patient cannot always understand the therapist.
3. *Global aphasia* is aphasia in its most extensive form and is caused by severe damage to the speech center. Patients suffering from global aphasia cannot speak, read, or write, and comprehend only a little.

For many patients, aphasia is temporary, or partial and responsive to treatment; however, treatment requires great patience and understanding. Dysarthria, a condition in which muscles needed for speech are affected, should not be confused with aphasia.

Assessment

There are a few simple procedures nursing personnel can use to assess aphasia and to complement the evaluation of the speech therapist. The care-giver should avoid tiring the patient. Can the patient say intelligible words in proper sequence? Can he understand what he hears, and respond to commands such as "hold up your hand?" Can he read? Can he name objects correctly? When making an assessment, keep the environment calm, the questions simple, and use positive reinforcement generously when he responds. From family or friends, it is often possible to determine the patient's native language, past education, and cultural background, and his present communicative ability. To aid in assessment, use nonverbal communication—touch, facial expression, and picture books, as well as the spoken word—anything that may help to establish communication.

Personal accounts, written by or about aphasic individuals, offer great insight into aphasia as well as specific guidelines for therapy. Understanding the subjective experience of aphasia is invaluable both for the patient's rehabilitation and for family counseling. A partial list of these accounts is included at the end of this chapter.

Although each case of aphasia is unique, there are some experiences common to most persons with aphasia. Some key points gleaned from two such accounts are included here.

Stroke

Those with aphasia as a result of stroke may react to their stroke with surprising calm at first. Moss reports that he felt almost no anxiety or concern for the first few weeks following his stroke because he had no inner thoughts.[4] He could not "speak" to himself about his situation. He writes, "It was as if the stroke benumbed any emotional investment in the future. . . ."[4] When recovery begins, this calm is replaced by great anxiety and frustration that may persist for years. Such temporary calmness *may* make early therapeutic efforts particularly difficult, since the patient is unmotivated.

Moss does complain about feeling that his physicians ignored his psychological state during his hospitalization. He was aware that they seemed interested only in his neurologic impairment and not at all in his psychological reaction to it. Even though he could not communicate at all, he was offended by this attitude.[4]

Recovery

Aphasic individuals relate that efforts to speak are extremely exhausting. It is a difficult and emotionally stressful task, and patients tire quickly. It is important to have patience, to be sensitive to this, and to avoid overtaxing the patient.

Another common characteristic of relearning speech is step progress. One week, improvement may be dramatic, and the next week, no progress may be made at all.

Moss described his experience: "This matter of recovery is an uncertain thing—it is an uphill struggle of a most uneven character."[4] Therapists need not be discouraged by learning plateaus.

Crowded and noisy rooms are especially difficult for people recovering from aphasia. It is arduous for them to follow one conversation in a room in which many conversations are taking place. Music, as well as other noises, may be a serious distraction. Speaking with a single person is less difficult than trying to follow a conversation that includes several people. Care-givers should, of course, always speak clearly and slowly.

Memory is affected as well as speech in most instances of aphasia. Certainly the two are interrelated. Knox reports that his wife's memory was selective after her stroke.[5] She recalled events of particular importance, but could not remember less significant occurrences. He surmises that there is some kind of memory threshold, which may be lower with aphasia; he suggests that this is a cause of spontaneous memory selection.[5] Moss[4] also reports a persistent loss of memory that extends beyond remembering certain words. Interestingly, he compares his memory to that of an old man; he feels that his stroke, in effect, aged him prematurely.[4] Therefore, inconsistent memory should be taken into consideration when caring for the aphasic individual.

Personality changes are not uncommon experiences. Because of the high level of anxiety and frustration, persons with aphasia sometimes become oversensitive and annoyed by minor problems. Understandably, they often experience bouts of severe depression and may even be temporarily suicidal. It is not uncommon for aphasic individuals to have great difficulty making decisions. Families of aphasic persons may benefit from understanding counsel to facilitate ways of coping with these changes.

According to Moss,[4] an occasional misuse of words may persist even after virtually total recovery. He writes that after 2 years, he still might ask his children if they want to go to the "antifreeze" rather than the Dairy Queen, or direct them to put on their BVDs instead of their pajamas. When rushed, he still may use a nonsense word. A telephone conversation is particularly trying for the individual.[4]

A final point: For some reason, aphasia tends to stimulate the use of profanity, causing the person to use offensive language without realizing it. It is a kind of nonsense speech. In other situations, profanity says it all:

> We never shall forget the 75-year-old woman who had a stroke and was attempting to express her emotional feelings about her suffering. She struggled mightily for a number of minutes but the words just would not come. Finally, everything momentarily fell into place and she shouted "Shit!" to the heavens, with a triumphant voice and a gleam in her eye—summing up her feelings succinctly. We and she alike considered it a therapeutic victory.[2]

Suggestions for Therapy

Evaluation by a speech therapist should be obtained before a plan of action is instituted. Much success has been reported with group therapy for aphasic patients. Small groups can be organized on units with no special facilities. Groups have been organized by nurses with no special knowledge of group therapy techniques. It is helpful to use brightly colored pictures and particular themes to stimulate casual conversation. Sharing of the experience of aphasia is another approach.

Another therapeutic technique is the use of memorization. One stroke patient discovered that although he could speak only haltingly, he could sing old, familiar songs perfectly. He subsequently found that memorizing songs, psalms, or poems aided his speech immensely.[6] "My speech took a great forward spurt. I seemed to gain as much in one week as I had previously in three months. . . . The speechless one was talking freely."[6] He suggests that memorization is a great aid to enlarging vocabulary.

Finally, the relationship between anxiety and rehabilitation cannot be overemphasized. Those with aphasia experience continual anxiety, both about their ability to communicate and about their lives in general. It is extremely difficult to regain self-confidence, and the individual commonly remains very anxious about particular kinds of personal contact (i.e., meeting strangers, talking with professional colleagues, etc.). Even when recovery seems complete, anxiety often persists. The aphasia raises doubts about his ability to support his family and arouses fear of future strokes.

This observation has direct application to speech therapy. One aphasic individual,[7] who achieved almost complete recovery and became head of a speech pathology department at a medical school, seriously challenges the traditional approach of speech therapy.

> Buck says he found no assistance whatsoever from direct vocabulary and language drills—the majority of his successes were almost wholly dependent upon his psychological security and the deletion of unrealistic pressures concerning word-by-word expression in conversation.[4]

The prime quality of recovery from aphasia is high personal motivation sustained by "spontaneous recovery," when a patient happens to hit on something that seems effective for him, Moss says.[4] Most speech therapy, he suggests, is able to accomplish only the most fundamental rehabilitation.[4] An open mind and the willingness to experiment—and encourage experimentation—are key values when working with aphasia.

REFERENCES

[1]American Foundation for the Blind: *An Introduction to Working with the Aging Person Who is Visually Handicapped.* New York, 1972

[2]Butler, R.N., and Lewis, M.I.: *Aging and Mental Health.* St. Louis: C.V. Mosby Co., 1973.

[3]Burnside, I.: *Psycho-Social Aspects of Aging.* New York: McGraw-Hill, 1973.

PERSONAL ACCOUNTS OF APHASIA

[4]Moss, C.: Recovery with Aphasia. Urbana: Univ. of Illinois Press, 1972.

[5]Knox, D.R.: Portrait of Aphasia. Detroit: Wayne State Univ. Press, 1971.

[6]Rose, R.H.: A physician's account of his own aphasia. *Speech Hear. Disord.* 13:294–305, 1948.

[7]Buck, M.: The language of disorders: A personal and professional account of aphasia. *J. Rehabil.* 29:37–38, 1963.

SUGGESTED READING

Boothroyd, A.: Technology and deafness. *Volta Review.* January, 1975, pp. 27–34.

Farrel, B: *Pat and Roald.* New York: Random House, 1969. (This is the account of the recovery of the actress Patricia Neal.)

Richie, D.: Stroke: *A Diary of Recovery.* London: Faber and Faber, 1966.

State of California, Dept. of Social Welfare: "Helping Individuals Adjust to Blindness." Program Guide No. 2, March 1968.

Chapter 6

Mental Disorders in Later Life

My anger, because I am old, is considered a sign of madness or senility. Is this not cruel? Are we to be deprived even of righteous anger? Is even irritability to be treated as a "symptom."

—M. Sarton[1]

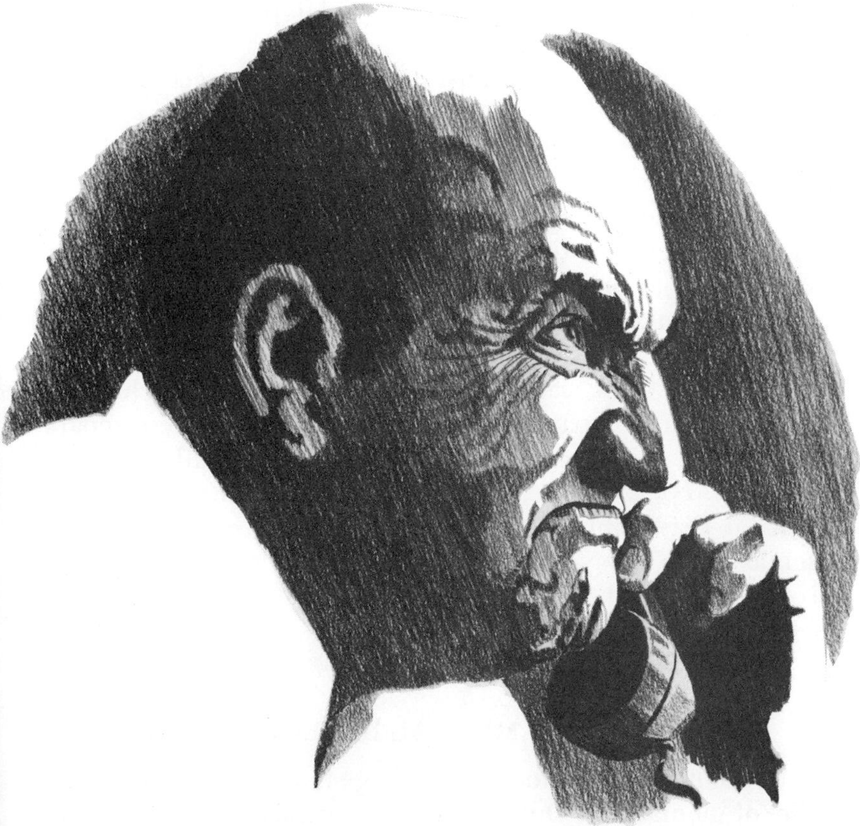

The subject of mental disorders among the elderly is extremely complex. On the most basic level, nursing personnel need to recognize genuine mental impairments as distinct from opinions that arise from stereotyped attitudes about the elderly.

> My anger, because I am old, is considered a sign of madness or senility. Is this not cruel? Are we to be deprived even of righteous anger? Is even irritability to be treated as a "symptom."[1]

Included on this level is an awareness of the myth of mental deterioration among the elderly.

On another level, it is important to be aware of the interaction of multiple psychiatric and physiological factors among aged patients. This interaction is particularly relevant to health care planning for the aged and is crucial to proper diagnosis of mental symptoms.

On yet a third level, we must deal with the subject of organic brain syndrome, found most often in the elderly.

These diseases may be either acute or chronic; distinguishing between the two is oftentimes difficult; and restorative care may be helpful, in degrees, for both conditions.

Finally, there are the functional (nonorganic) mental disorders. Many old people (a conservative estimate is 15%)[2] suffer from functional disorders, and nurses encounter these problems in virtually every health care setting.

For purposes of clarity, we will discuss these four levels of mental disorder separately. In reality, of course, these separations do not exist; patients may have any combination of these problems. For example, an ill, confused patient may find that even his reasonable feelings and thoughts are interpreted as "senile"; also, a person with organic brain syndrome may suffer from a functional disorder as well.

THE MYTH OF MENTAL DETERIORATION

Part of our social mythology of old age is a belief in the inevitability of mental loss. Our prevailing cultural expectation is that aging is accompanied by decline of mental abilities and that this decline is irreversible. Not only does this attitude increase each person's fear of growing old, but it also leads us to react in a predetermined way to confusion and inappropriate behavior in elderly patients. Professional education in itself does not free us of this cultural bias.

> One woman of 91 was hospitalized for a fractured hip. For days after her admission, she muttered continually to all staff, "I *wish* I hadn't left that banana on the windowsill." No one understood the remark, and many thought she was confused. Finally, one concerned nurse visited the patient's home, but found no banana. Talking to the landlady, she discovered that the landlady had thrown away a banana that she had found on the windowsill while cleaning.
>
> When the nurse returned to the hospital, she asked the patient why she was so anxious about the banana. The patient replied that she was afraid it would rot and attract flies and that someone would decide that she couldn't return home because she couldn't do her housekeeping.

In fact, structural and physical changes do occur in the brain in later life. Loss of neurons takes place throughout life, and the accumulated loss is an inevitable aspect of aging. Studies indicate that there is 33.3% neuron loss from young adulthood to very old age (65–80). The rate of loss, however, varies widely from person to person.

Even more important to nursing care, the functional meaning of neuron loss varies as well. Neurophysical evidence of brain impairment is very prevalent in the elderly, *even in those with no apparent mental deterioration.* Neuronal loss does not necessarily mean poor functioning, as we have far more neurons than we ever use. The reverse is also true: Confusion and erratic behavior in elderly patients is not always due to loss of neurons or other brain tissue change and, very often, is neither irreversible nor untreatable.

Most research on the subject of changes in intelligence over the life span has used intelligence tests. These studies emphasize that differences within groups of elderly people are frequently as large as, or larger than, differences between the elderly and younger control groups. In some early tests comparing different age groups to estimate changes over the years, the results indicated peak performance during the late teens and early 20s. Other tests, concerned with the performance of the same individual at different ages, indicate peak capability around the age of 50; later declines in performance were still significantly higher than results recorded at age 22. Overall, though test results vary and intelligence tests themselves are a much criticized analytic tool, intelligence testing has led to two salient conclusions: age affects various abilities differently (speed of response most commonly declines in later years), and individual differences merit much more attention than age group variation.

In testing done with learning ability and memory, dramatic improvement in elderly subjects was observed if the presentation of the test material was slowly paced, or if subjects were allowed to respond at their own rate. Learning ability is not normally impaired although the speed of response often declines. Other studies emphasize that emotional stress or poor health adversely affect performance on learning tests. This relationship between stress and mental capability—common to all ages—is particularly crucial in the elderly.

The aged are as aware as anyone of the myth about mental deterioration, so they respond to any sign of loss of mental ability with great anxiety. Especially in the hospital, the clinical environment coupled with such a profound sense of loss may be overwhelming. The first sign of mental impairment, such as loss of recent memory or confusion, is often less of a problem than the patient's reaction to it. It is another case of self-fulfilling prophecy. The anxiety aroused by the patient's own awareness of his inability, though it may be temporary, may lead to such severe stress that more psychic and physical damage follows. *The myth of mental deterioration affects the elderly more drastically than anyone else.* When we realize that this fear often follows earlier losses of income, status, self-esteem, perhaps home and spouse, we can understand it when we encounter desperation or hopelessness. Supportive, reassuring care is essential.

The effects of interaction of multiple factors are demonstrated in the following case report.

> Mr. B., a former executive, at 78 was hospitalized for depression because he "couldn't think of anything more to do." Therapy directed him toward long-postponed activities, and he improved rapidly and was sent home. A few months later, he was hospitalized for a mild myocardial infarction. He was placed on digitalis, diuretics, and a low-salt diet, and was told to restrict his physical activity.
>
> At home, he ate almost nothing because he heartily disliked the low-salt diet, but continued to take diuretics as directed. Within a few weeks, he was lethargic, drowsy, and extremely dizzy. Again, he was hospitalized. As a result of his diet and diuretic therapy, Mr. B. developed fluid and electrolyte depletion and consequent orthostatic hypotension, with some actual, though reversible, mental impairment.
>
> On a normal diet and without diuretics, he regained his appetite and energy. This time, when he was sent home, he was encouraged to be physically active, and continued on digitalis therapy with only intermittent diuretic therapy.[3]

Mr. B. is an example of the way in which multiple factors interact in elderly patients. A patient may begin as a psychiatric patient and suddenly suffer a heart attack, or drug therapies for physical complaints may lead to deteriorated mental capacities. The interrelationship of psychic and physiological factors is critical in geriatrics.

A number of physical diseases commonly present themselves *first* through mental disorientation in the aged. This is further complicated by the fact that elderly patients often fail to report physical symptoms accurately. One useful generality is that mental disorientation accompanying physical disease is often irregular. Confusion comes and goes, and is punctuated with periods of normal clarity. Such a waxing and waning pattern should be carefully noted. Sudden changes in mental state may indicate physical disease as well.

Some conditions notorious for their impact on reasoning ability are highlighted in Table 6.1. Cardiovascular disease often leads to confusion because, in older patients, even comparatively small declines in optimal blood flow to the brain can impair mental ability. In later years, cardiac output is much decreased, and perfusion volume to the brain declines year by year. Practically all metabolic disorders can appear first as mental aberrations.

Drug therapies may be an insidious cause of disorientation in an older patient.

> One man of 63 became incoherent when he entered the hospital with a broken. back. The nurses speculated that his son was sneaking alcohol to him. They looked the patient over suspiciously every time the son came to visit, incidentally making him markedly uncomfortable. This misdirected guesswork delayed the discovery that it was not contraband alcohol at all, but a toxic reaction to a prescribed medication.

Drug tolerances are notably lower in old age, and effective dosage levels are often very close to toxicity levels. The central nervous system frequently reacts first.

Table 6.1. Conditions Known for Impact on Reasoning Ability

Disease state	Mental reaction
Myxedema Pneumonia Prostatism with urinary retention	Confusion may be first sign
Cardiovascular disorders Cerebrovascular accident Cardiac disease Cardiac arrhythmias Myocardial infarction Congestive heart failure	May cause confusion without chest pain (Cardiac arrhythmias, Myocardial infarction) Mood change may appear before clinical symptoms
Metabolic disorders Diabetes Thyroid hypofunction or hyperfunction Uremia Compromise of liver function	Mental changes may be first symptom (Thyroid hypofunction or hyperfunction)
Hematologic disorders Iron-deficiency anemia Pernicious anemia Folic acid deficiency	

Two types of drugs, especially, should be observed with utmost care. Tranquilizers, sedatives and antidepressants may intensify mental problems rather than ameliorate them. Drugs commonly used in treatment of cardiovascular disease (such as digitalis, diuretics, and antihypertensive agents) often trigger serious problems. Diuretics may alter the electrolyte balance, already sensitive in older patients; digitalis can directly affect the central nervous system; and antihypertensive medication can decrease cerebral blood flow. Determining the cause of disorientation in a medicated older patient is like a Gordian knot—is it a drug, or the disease itself? Older patients and all others concerned should be told as much as possible about the mental side effects to be expected from either the disease or the medication.

Just as mental impairment may be a leading symptom of physical disease, physical health is the most important factor relevant to psychiatric disorders. In one psychiatric hospital sample, 80% of the patients suffered from physical illness serious enough to require supervision.[4]

ORGANIC BRAIN SYNDROME

Distinct from disorientation caused by disease in other body systems, mental disorder may be due to organic brain syndrome, caused by damage to the function of brain tissue. The type and seriousness of the mental symptoms is *not* necessarily related to the extent of brain damage. Just the opposite is true: Wide variation is to be expected, influenced by virtually all the other variables in the patient's life. Brain damage is not the sole determining factor, and patients with organic brain syndrome may respond well to treatment.

The characteristic symptoms of organic brain syndrome include disorientation in time, place, and person; memory defects; and difficulty in problem-solving, comprehension, and judgment. Usually emotional reactions are easily triggered and extreme. (None of these symptoms are restricted to organic brain syndrome. Other conditions may be responsible for extreme disorientation.)

Questions such as "Where are we?" "What month is it?" "When were you born?" may be useful for broad evaluations of a patient's capacities. Questioning, however, can be unreliable. Other variables, such as emotional responses to the questioning, deafness, or decline in speed of response can affect the patient's response.

Organic brain syndrome may be chronic and permanent or acute and reversible. An acute state may lead to chronic functional disorders due to severe anxiety and depression.

Chronic Organic Brain Syndrome

The two most common chronic forms of organic brain syndrome are associated with degenerative brain disease or cerebral arteriosclerosis. Severity may range from barely perceptible symptoms to profound loss of function. These conditions may be further complicated by psychotic, neurotic, or behavioral disorders. Senility may also be related to genetic factors or to a slow virus. These are *not* normal conditions of aging but constitute distinct brain disease.

Several methods are available to determine the extent of organic brain damage. Normally, diagnosis relies on one or a combination of four procedures: (1) electroencephalography, (2) determining cerebral blood flow pattern by a method involving inhalation of 133-xenon, (3) echoencephalography, and (4) brain scanning. These methods are most useful when used together.

It is often difficult to differentiate between organic brain syndrome and depressive states. Some investigators[2] feel that organic senile psychosis is itself a functional state brought about by accumulated stresses of aging. Clearly, the distinction between functional and organic disorders is often unclear.

Acute Organic Brain Syndrome

The most common indication of acute (reversible) organic brain syndrome is a *fluctuating* level of awareness, orientation or memory. Behavior may include restlessness, dazed expression, aggressiveness, and sometimes delusions and severe anxiety. Thirteen percent of acute instances of organic brain syndrome are caused by congestive heart failure.[2] Malnutrition (especially vitamin B_{12} or folic acid deficiency), anemia, infection, cerebrovascular accidents, drugs and other toxic substances, head trauma, alcohol—all may cause acute states. Other causes are postural hypotension, hormonal imbalances, extracranial carotid disease, or normal pressure hydrocephalus. Older people are likely to be more vulnerable than younger people to exhaustion, vitamin deficiencies, and general disease.

Many laymen and too many medical personnel refer to chronic brain syndrome with the emotion-laden term of senile. Acute conditions are too often confused with chronic states and considered untreatable. Differentiation between the two—in diagnosis and treatment—began only 30 or 40 years ago. Chronic brain syndrome is irreversible, but even though brain damage is permanent, many emotional and physical symptoms can be treated with reality orientation and other techniques. Functioning often can be supported and improved.

Restorative Nursing

Restorative nursing embraces several techniques that benefit individuals suffering from either form of organic brain syndrome. All these interventions are designed to maintain contact with reality. They can be used in all settings, in formalized groups and in informal interaction.

Social therapy. Converse with the patient, and encourage him to relate to others.

Work therapy. Provide simple, productive handiwork opportunities.

Play and games. Play simple games, and plan recreational activities.

Movement and exercise therapy. Encourage the patient to move actively and to exercise all his limbs.

Reality orientation. This important approach encompasses many techniques, all geared to improving the individual's orientation. Large clocks and calendars are often helpful for time orientation, and conspicuous signs are valuable for place orientation. One example is brightly painted footprints on the floor leading to the bathrooms or the dining room. Inventiveness is the key. Reality orientation may also include organized programs in which the nursing staff presents the patient with basic personal information, beginning with his name, the place, and the date. Instruction progresses to other facts, such as his age, home town, and former occupation, after the first level has been mastered. It is helpful to reality orientation if the confusing elements of hospital routine are minimized.

Behavior modification. Aimed at changing specific negative or dysfunctional behavior, this technique usually requires that the staff predetermine a consistent response to a particular behavior problem.

> One old resident in an intensive care facility was extremely anxious. He constantly repeated, "When's dinner, Mrs. ?" "Can I have a cigarette, Mrs.?" That is all he would say. Staff decided to repeat his questions to him: "When *is* dinner?" When he discovered he could answer his own questions, the questioning gradually ceased. Other interactions followed, and soon his anxiety was much less pronounced.[5]

Behavior modification also may involve appropriate rewards for desirable behavior.

Drug Therapy

Psychotherapeutic agents are often administered to patients with organic brain syndrome. Sedatives and tranquilizers may be needed to control the behavior of severely brain-damaged patients. These drugs should always be used with care, since drug tolerances in the aged are usually low. Other therapeutic approaches may complement the use of these drugs whenever possible.

FUNCTIONAL DISORDERS

The American Psychiatric Association estimated, in 1971, that 15% of the older population needed mental health services.

Butler[4] considers this a conservative estimate. Many factors contribute to mental stress in the elderly, especially institutionalization, chronic disorders, both physical and mental, poverty, and the low self-esteem and lack of social contact characteristic of the aged in our society. In addition, the experience of normal aging and of coming to terms with death often taxes the coping mechanisms of many. The elderly commonly experience anxiety, loneliness, and grief. They may suffer guilt, rage, and a sense of helplessness. Adequate outlets for these emotions are difficult to find.

Khanlari, a Persian poet, captures some of this feeling superbly:

> Sorrowful grew the eagle's spirit
> and heart when he beheld the
> season of youth depart. Far, far
> away: when he perceived his turn
> was nigh to end, the sun's last
> radiance burn the roof-edge of
> his life.[6]

The most prevalent functional disorders among the aged are depression, paranoia, and schizophrenia. Depression, in particular, is more frequent and intense in old age. There are two main groups of elderly psychiatric patients, those who have been chronically ill for many years, and those who first develop mental disorders in later life. Individuals in the first group may have been institutionalized for a long period of time.

Depression

Depression is usually manifested by feelings of sadness, helplessness, lack of vitality, and low self-regard. Individuals may be extremely withdrawn. They may appear confused and rarely speak. Delusions, memory loss, and disorientation, often assumed to be organically based, are frequently secondary symptoms of depression. Depression is often manifested in physical symptoms as well: sleeplessness, loss of appetite, fatigue, and constipation. Hypochondriasis is common.

Loneliness, rejection, physical disease, and grief all may contribute to depression. Fear of death may intensify mental stress.

Many depressed patients, hospitalized for years, may originally have been mistakenly institutionalized after experiencing grief and shock. Their feelings of rejection and isolation result in extreme withdrawal from their environment.

Paranoia

Suspiciousness, insecurity, and anxiety characterize paranoia. Delusions are typical. Symptoms may be generalized or discrete. In old age, paranoid delusions are often directed toward someone spatially or emotionally close (rather than remote and powerful distant forces, more common to younger people). Deafness contributes to paranoia, as does the clinical environment itself for some people. Paranoia is often short-term and treatable.

Schizophrenia

A chronic mental disorder sometimes associated with chronic brain syndrome, schizophrenia occurs at both psychotic and neurotic levels. Hallucinations, delusions, and poor results on reality testing are characteristic. Rarely is it newly developed in old age; it is more likely to occur in the elderly as a long-term chronic disorder.

Hypochondriasis

A special problem to nursing personnel, hypochondriasis is often a symptom of depression, but may occur alone. It may be a means of attaining interaction with others or a way to displace anxiety or the expression of an inner sense of deterioration. Sometimes hypochondriasis serves as a self-punishment for guilt feelings or as an aid in achieving control over others. An unpublished paper on "crocks" suggests that hypochondriac individuals seek help in order to avoid more serious mental illness.[7] Care-giving may be, in itself, a preventive measure, especially if it can lead the patient to an awareness of the real reasons for seeking help. "Anxiety should be listened to and accepted."[4]

REMOTIVATION

Remotivation and resocialization programs have had remarkable success with depressed, withdrawn elderly patients. Remotivation is the first step in the rehabilitative process, and can be one part of a comprehensive resocialization program.

This approach is designed for long-term, chronic psychiatric patients and for use in extended care facilities and nursing homes. Any effort to encourage social participation, such as arts, crafts, or recreational group activities, is therapeutic, but care should be taken to avoid infantalism.

Butler emphasizes five steps in the remotivation technique[4]:

1. The climate of acceptance—establishing a warm friendly relationship in the group
2. A bridge to reality—reading, or objective poetry, current events, *etc*.
3. Sharing the world—development of topics introduced in step 2 through planned objective questions, use of props, *etc*.
4. An appreciation of the work of the world—designed to stimulate the patients to think about work in relation to themselves
5. The climate of appreciation—expression of enjoyment at getting together, *etc*.

Remotivation is directed to the healthy aspect of each patient rather than to his sickness, on a round-the-clock basis.*

Human[8] has described an extremely effective resocialization program in a state hospital ward with 60 severely regressed, elderly female patients. Nurses were the prime initiators of this program. The major objectives were rehabilitation, resocialization, and the placement of the patient in the community. It is significant that these goals are directed to rehumanizing the patients' lives and revitalizing their ability to cope with life, *not* to restructuring personality.

The staff was depressed and unhappy by the ward environment.[8] They decided, with administrative support, to restructure the entire health care program. Beginning with a 5-day sensitivity type program for staff, the resocialization program included the following steps: (1) a change of physical environment, with bright colors, a coffee urn, no uniforms, and new clothing for patients; (2) group nursing, in which each patient was assigned to a particular staff member; (3) remotivation groups, led by nurses and focusing on such topics as gardening, sewing, current events, or travel (these groups included snacks); (4) patient independence and interaction, through the use of a buddy system, the improvement of personal appearances, recreational trips to neighborhood parks, musical activities, etc.; and (5) a special emphasis on careful discharge planning.[8] Relatives and friends were encouraged to participate, and the help of young people from the local Neighborhood Youth Corps was invaluable.

Perhaps most importantly, the attitude of the staff was one "of hopeful expectancy for patient improvement."[8] This attitude was conveyed to the patients, and they responded. The program had a tremendous impact on staff morale, lightened the physical workload, and decreased the patients' reliance on drugs. The staff began to function as a cohesive therapeutic team.

> The rewards of meaningful nursing programs of this kind are twofold because both staff and patients have a positive rather than a negative attitude toward the prognosis of the elderly psychotic person.[8]

REFERENCES

[1]Sarton, M.: *As We Are Now.* New York: W. W. Norton & Company, Inc., 1973.

[2]Butler, R.N., and Lewis, M.I.: *Aging and Mental Health.* St. Louis: C.V. Mosby, 1973.

[3]Busse, E.W., and Pfeiffer, E.: *Mental Illness in Later Life.* Washington, D.C.: American Psychiatric Association, 1973.

[4]Simon, A.: "The Psychology of Aging." In *Aging: Prospects and Issues.* Los Angeles: Ethel Percy Andrus Gerontology Center, Univ. of Southern California, 1973.

[5]Tyberg, D.: Personal interview, Dec. 16, 1975.

[6]Khanlari: "The Eagle." in *Persian Poems.* Edited by A.J. Arberry. London: Everyman's Library, 1960, p. 141.

[7]Myersberg, A., et al: Unpublished work. Washington, D.C.: George Washington Univ. Medical School, 1966.

[8]Human, M.E.: "The Aged Psychiatric Patient." In *Psycho-Social Nursing Care of the Aged.* Edited by I.M. Burnside. New York: McGraw-Hill, 1973.

*Remotivation kits for nursing homes and mental hospitals are available through the American Psychiatric Association, Washington, D.C.

SUGGESTED READING

Curtin, S.R.: Nobody Ever Dies of Old Age. Boston, Mass.: Little, Brown and Company, 1972.

Chapter 7

Caring for the Dying Person

Doctor, Doctor, will I die?
Yes, my child, and so will I.

—Anonymous

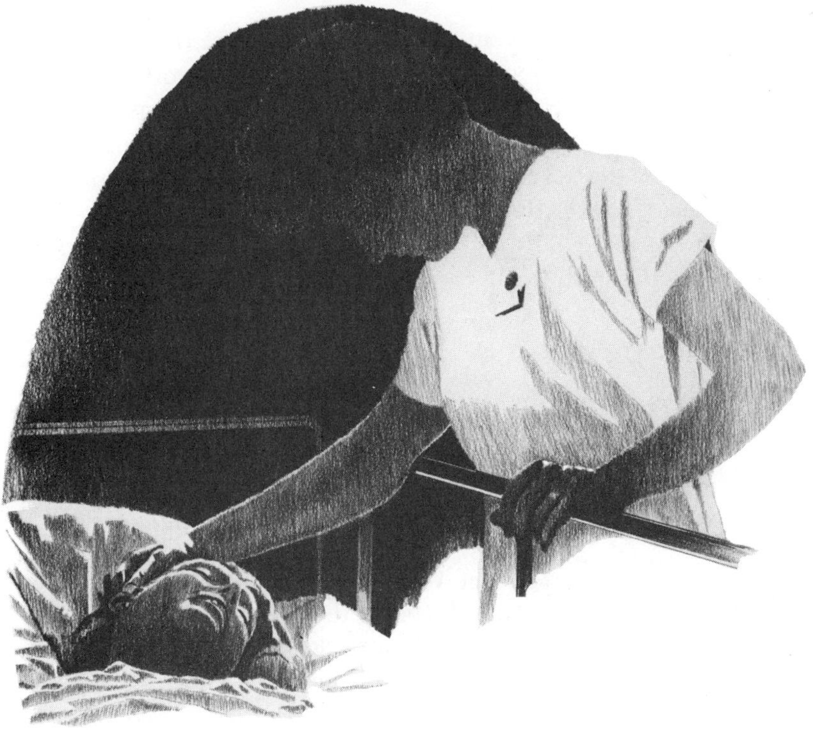

DEATH IN AMERICAN CULTURE

It is commonplace to say that Americans strive to ignore death. Our culture places premium value on strength, progress, and youth. We tend to devalue old age, and death—a "morbid" subject—is taboo. It is referred to euphemistically, isolated in hospitals and nursing homes, and carefully concealed by both hospital procedure and morticians.

This attitude toward death is detrimental to the dying, to their families, and to care-givers. It provides no guidelines or cultural wisdom, and is too often manifested in individual relationships as well: Our cultural denial of death leads to neglect of the dying.

Yet this view of death-denial in America, true as it is, is superficial. We daily cope with death and respond to dying with the full range of emotion that all humanity brings to this final, profound event. Our cultural attitude does not shield us from death, but it does impinge on our reaction. It is important only because it makes dying so difficult.

This is especially true in our time. Benjamin Franklin approached death with humor and confidence, as his epitaph shows:

The Body of
B. Franklin, Printer,
(Like the Cover of an Old Book
Its Contents torn out
And stript of its Lettering & Gilding)
Lies here, Food for Worms.
But the Work shall not be lost;
For it will, (as he believ'd) appear once more
In a new and more elegant Edition
Revised and corrected
By the Author.

The modern changes in our institutions and in our religious beliefs leave us, all too often, bereft of a system of meaning with which to respond to death. Our theological doctrines are now often questioned, and science is actively redirecting the process of dying. It is the transitional nature of our present society that renders dying so difficult, more so than any entrenched attitude of denial. The denial is really an expression of our confusion and fear.

In more traditional cultures, death is often accepted gracefully as a part of life. Rituals of death may be the cause for village celebration. In Bali in Indonesia, for example, the (usually) elaborate cremation rites are followed by feasts; the religion of the Balinese includes the concept of reincarnation, and they see death as part of a process of rebirth and renewal. Traditional peoples may be so accepting of death that the aged are able to choose the time of their own dying.

Kubler-Ross relates the story of an old Eskimo woman, old Sarah, who summoned her minister, family, and friends 3 weeks before her death to come worship with her. As soon as all were gathered, services were said, her gifts distributed, and her farewells made, she quietly died.[1] Osceola, the great Seminole chief was able to rise before his death, don his full ceremonial dress, smilingly bid farewell to his family and friends, and die gladly with his war-knife clasped across his chest.

This capacity to accept death willingly is not limited to others. There are numerous reports of Americans who have died at their chosen time. Kubler-Ross mentions her husband's elderly uncle who lingered in his dying until he found an opportunity to be of help to her. She sprained her ankle, and he gave her his cane, saying he would no longer need it. He died an hour later.[1] Customarily, this kind of death is not permitted in America.

In this chapter, we will consider what *is* permitted to the dying in America, examine the difficulties of dying in an institution, and propose ways the care-givers can help.

There can be no genuine help for the dying without constant realization that here is one of man's fundamental mysteries. There is a perpetual and profound conflict between the peaceful acceptance of inevitable death and life's struggle against it. This contradiction permeates the care we are able to give. There is no resolution, beyond the fact that the choice belongs to the dying person.

Finally, our capacity to give care depends, in large part, on our own feelings about death. Consider this old story:

> A servant went to the market in Baghdad and met Death there. He saw Death reach for him as he passed. He raced home, and begged his master to give him a horse and money so that he could flee to Samarra "where Death cannot find me." His master agreed, and he galloped off.
>
> Later, his master went to the market and was surprised to find Death there. "Why did you jump at my servant?" he asked.
>
> Death replied, "I didn't jump. I only started with surprise to find him here in Baghdad when I have an appointment with him tonight in Samarra."

If we are trying to run like the servant to Samarra, we will not be there to help our patients meet death.

NURSING CARE FOR THE DYING PERSON

The first concern of nursing the dying person is the recognition of the individuality of each patient. Each person brings to dying his unique system of belief, feeling, and attitude, and it is through a respect for the integrity of each personality that care-giving is made possible. The dying need to have recognition of their uniqueness, or their care will be depersonalizing and mechanical. A deeply religious person may feel quite differently about death than a person who does not believe in God. A person who has experienced pain and poor health for many years may feel differently than one suddenly struck with illness. In fact, each individual approaches death along his own path, and care-givers must go *there* to reach him. The nursing focus is always on the individual. Consider the thoughts of one woman, Dorothy, aged 75, a dying patient in a nursing home:

> I stepped out into the night. My night. It was black night and the stars were my stars. I was alone with them. It was so still, the only sound was the tide coming, coming in, coming in. It was a pulse, it was there, it never stopped. It said be still and know that I am here. The timing of the pulse was the timing of my pulse. So I am the child of the tide.[1]

In discussing our knowledge of dying and the care of the dying, it is unavoidable to employ generalizations. It is understood that these ideas serve *only* to supplement a recognition of each individual.

The Five Stages of Dying

Kubler-Ross outlined five stages a patient experiences in coping with dying.[2] It is emphasized that not all patients pass through every stage, nor do they all conform to this sequence. The five stages are only a conceptual framework to aid in the understanding of a patient's feelings; gleaned from Kubler-Ross's extensive work with dying patients. Very briefly:

1. Denial. The initial reaction to knowledge of impending death is commonly some form of denial. How denial is expressed depends on the past life pattern of the person. The degree of denial often depends on how the patient has been told, how much time he has to prepare, and how he has coped with stressful situations in the past. Some people maintain their denial until death.
2. Anger. Resentment and envy of the living often follow denial. This anger explodes in many directions, toward family, physician, nursing staff, and others. Kubler-Ross feels that it is helpful to allow the patient control over his situation whenever possible, since loss of control aggravates this anger.[2]
3. Bargaining. A patient may express the desire to do one last act, or he may engage in "deals" with God. These bargains take many forms, and may not seem rational to onlookers. Kubler-Ross's famous story concerns a woman who asked to be allowed only to attend her son's forthcoming wedding. Returning triumphant to the hospital, she said: "Don't forget, Dr. Ross, I have another son!"[2] Of course, the expressed wishes of the dying should be granted whenever possible.
4. Depression. The dying often experience a period of profound sadness and withdrawal. This depression is a form of preparatory grief, and this grief must be worked through to enable the individual to pass on to the final stage of the dying process. He may ask for fewer visitors, to be left alone; the patient's wishes should take prece-

dence over those of others. His family may need special help to understand and accept this behavior.

5. Acceptance. With time and help, acceptance is the prelude to a peaceful death. Although the dying patient may be withdrawn and quiet at this stage, it is essential that he not be abandoned. He still needs companionship and support. Paul Ramsey, a theologian, believes, "The sting of death is solitude. Desertion is more choking than death and more feared."[3]

Listening

How can nurses help the dying person as he experiences these feelings? The key skill needed is the ability to listen. A nurse who herself was once close to death has written that listening and the willingness to talk about death are more important than anything else.[4] She says that the physical presence of another and the opportunity to share one's feelings are the primary needs of a dying patient.[4]

Listening requires that nurses be aware of their own feelings about death so they may frankly discuss dying with a patient. An honest appraisal of our own feelings, our fears and biases, is prerequisite to caring for a dying patient. Only then can we distinguish between our own feelings and those of our patient.

Listening also requires the ability to listen for clues that a dying person wants to share his thoughts. Kubler-Ross reports over and over again that the dying patients she interviewed expressed great relief and pleasure at the opportunity to talk about dying.[1] Families often avoid direct discussion, and physicians may also be reluctant to talk with their dying patients. It is the nurse, who spends the most time with the patient and who may be the most accessible, to whom the patient looks for companionship.

Management of the Dying Patient

A six-point nursing plan for the dying patient has been proposed.[5] The general outline hinges on an understanding of the needs just discussed: (1) First of all, a nurse must recognize and work to resolve her own feelings about death. (2) She must talk and listen when the patient indicates, verbally or nonverbally, the desire to communicate, hopefully long before death. (3) She must help each patient to live until he dies, recognizing that dying is an integral part of life. (4) The nurse tries to understand what the patient is experiencing, and accepts the patient's feelings. (5) She does her best to guarantee that the patient will feel like an important individual, whether or not he can be helped, and she grants him the right to decision-making. (6) She does not desert the patient. Although at times there is little or no need for words, companionship is still needed until death ensues.

Once the nurse has learned to work *with* the aged dying patient in this way, care is directed to four major needs: (1) freedom from pain, (2) freedom from loneliness, (3) conservation of energy, and (4) maintenance of self-esteem. These four, interwoven into the care-giving process, are the primary nursing goals.

Freedom from pain. The aged dying patient usually experiences *chronic* pain rather than *acute* pain. Whereas acute pain, limited in duration, can be relieved by analgesics given on time and by other physical measures, chronic pain goes on and on. It does not improve or subside and may come to occupy the whole attention of the patient. Concern with withholding medication to prevent addiction is not appropriate for the chronic pain of a dying person. For chronic pain, the goal is to administer appropriate medication regularly, on time, and around the clock to give the patient maximum comfort. This procedure often eliminates the need for ever-increasing amounts of medication, and can allow the patient to retain clear consciousness.

Psychic pain compounds physical pain. Nursing actions include alleviating the pain of anxiety and sadness by being near, touching, sitting close by, listening, and demonstrating personal concern. Diversions such as backrubs, or the use of TV or radio may also help to ease psychic pain for a time.

Freedom from loneliness. Detached, mechanical care and a dim, hushed single room increase the patient's feelings of isolation and loneliness. These feelings may develop into fears. The dying patient needs a homelike environment, with bright colors, adequate light, and his personal possessions about him. A room located near activity is preferable to one at the "end of the hall." Visiting at any hour should be permitted the dying. In some situations, a nighttime "sitter" to provide emotional support is needed.

The nurse can do a great deal to alleviate loneliness by taking the time to sit and listen. Reminiscing is important to the dying patient as a way of reviewing his life, and it should not be shut off. Helping the patient to take walks or wheelchair rides also diminishes loneliness.

In St. Christopher's Hospice, in England, rooms with four patients are used very successfully to combat isolation. The routine practice of placing the dying patient in a single room deserves reexamination. Roommates can provide a large measure of support and companionship for each other.

It should be noted that some people desire solitude, and their wishes, too, should be respected.

Conservation of energy. This is, perhaps, the most tangible need of the dying patient, but freedom from pain and loneliness are prerequisites. The nurse is the manager of the dying person's energy resources. She must determine which activities are most important for him to continue—such as eating by himself, washing, receiving visitors, etc.—and which she can perform for him. These decisions need to be made with the patient's knowledge and participation, for care without explanation produces anxiety. All interventions to reduce anxiety help the patient to accumulate more usuable energy.

Maintenance of self-esteem. All these three activities contribute to this fourth major goal. The aged dying person often begins to feel out-of-place, unwanted, a "burden." Nurses can help the patient continue to respect and value himself until death by showing *their* respect. (Conversely, if they show no respect or baby the patient, they can effectively undermine the patient's remaining self-esteem.)

Interventions should be founded on respect and helpfulness. Care should be taken to avoid fostering feelings of dependency, guilt, or conflict. Maintaining the patient's best personal appearance and comfort will help to support self-esteem. Focusing attention on present satisfactions and opportunities for satisfaction in the near future may be more beneficial than continual emphasis on the past. Finally, self-esteem depends, in part, on the maintenance of meaningful social contact. The nurse tries to protect such relationships, as well as to involve herself in relationship with the patient.

The needs of elderly institutionalized patients require attention also.[4] These people, too, need ways to prepare for death. In a nursing home environment, it may be difficult to recognize when a patient wishes to ready himself for death. Some behavioral clues are useful to help nurses initiate assistance. When a person acts to distribute his possessions, or wishes to see clergy or people he hasn't seen in some time, a nurse is alerted to the fact that these patients may wish to prepare for dying.

Expectation of death is prevalent among elderly institutionalized people. Interviews of 54 alert, nonbedridden women in a nursing home, aged 65-85, were conducted to learn what they expected for themselves in 5 years' time[5]. Forty replied, in one way or another, that they expected to be dead.

Suicide and self-destructive behavior, such as refusing medication and food and risking danger, increases with age, especially in men. Self-destructive behavior can sometimes be discouraged by appropriate intervention. A careful patient history is the first step in setting realistic goals for care, according to one investigator.[5] Stress should be diminished whenever possible by keeping nursing assignments stable or by postponing moves. A communicative atmosphere may enable patients to express and work through their feelings about suicide and death.

Potentially suicidal persons need a protective environment and nursing care to counter their anguish. Depressed patients may respond well to kindness and empathy and to a concerted effort to interest them in activities. An assessment of a patient's recent losses, changes in health, or reminders of past grief may provide ideas for therapy. "No matter how self-destructive a man may be today, tommorow he may be deeply grateful for the fact that his feelings were respected but not obeyed."[6]

The use of pain-killers is needlessly controversial in the care of the dying. Surely the withholding of narcotics to avoid addiction is not as crucial as insuring the maximum comfort of the dying patient. Although many medications are commonly prescribed on a *pro re nata* basis, some nurses tend to increase the suffering of their patients through unnecessary delays.

The experimental use of LSD as a pain killer for terminal patients suggests that this drug may be more effective as an analgesic than most morphine derivatives. LSD (100 mg) is reported to relieve pain for 92 hours on the average, as opposed to 2–3 hours for morphine.[7] The drug has also been used, with mixed success, to aid patients in adjusting to terminal illness.[7] The use of LSD always requires very close supervision.

Sharing information with dying patients. Controversy continues about the wisdom of telling a person that he is dying. Nurses may find themselves trapped between the decision of the doctor and the expressed wishes of the patient. Unfortunately, although there is no simple solution to this question, the "conspiracy of silence" that often results isolates the dying person from genuine human contact.

Medical World News reported that 69–90% of the physicians queried were opposed to telling a patient that his illness was probably terminal.[8] In contrast, it is reported that 82% of terminal patients studied want to know the nature and severity of their illness.[8] This discrepancy places nurses in the terrible position of having to accommodate the physician rather than the patient.

There is, however, considerable evidence that a patient is usually aware of impending death even when he has not been informed. He may "feel it in his bones," or respond to nonverbal clues such as silence, distance, and the solemn faces of his visitors. Another reported study conducted in the late 1950s and early 1960s indicated that most dying patients know the truth and wish to discuss it.[8]

According to Kubler-Ross, the question ought to be not "Should I tell?" but "How should I share this knowledge with my patient?"[2] She stresses that it is crucial to leave the patient some reason to hope for recovery. Hope, she claims, enables the patient to retain confidence in his care, to be reassured that everything possible will be done for him, that he will not be "dropped."[2]

When a patient has been informed of the severity of his illness, he may wish to talk about dying with his family and nurses, and the nursing staff can facilitate these exchanges openly. Even when the patient has not been informed, a nurse can still offer a listening ear and a reassuring presence.

HELPING THE SURVIVORS

Nursing practitioners now feel responsible for helping the family of a dying patient as well as the patient himself. Polite evasion or preoccupation with other matters are no longer acceptable approaches, if they ever were. Needed communication does not conflict with visible physical care; both are priority nursing activities.

The pattern of grief discussed in Chapter 2 is often apparent in the feelings of family and friends. Numbness and denial may be a first reaction, followed by deep shock and distress.

In counseling a grieving family, the tool of listening is as useful as it is with the patient himself. Gentle questions help to continue a therapeutic flow of conversation. Families may need to know that anger and guilt are common and necessary expressions of grief. They may need support in dealing with the anger or withdrawn grief of their loved one. Giving them the opportunity to express their fears and feelings will make them more at ease in the institutional environment and will help them achieve rapport with nursing staff.

Family members may exhibit denial as much as patients. It should be respected and understood in the same way, as a part of working through their grief. Patients, however, may need to be protected from severe denial feelings in their families. One man suffered more from the feeling of disappointing his family than from the prospect of his own death. It may be possible to help a family avoid burdening their loved one with unrealistic plans and expectations.

Family members may bargain as well. In a sense, they may experience the dying process empathetically. They, too, may need companionship and understanding.

Give family members a role in the care of the patient. Encouraging them to help with oral care, feeding, or baths relieves nursing pressures while it gives the family an outlet for their feelings. However, families should not be forced into care roles. They will appreciate all the information you can give them about the patient's care and comfort.

When death is imminent, the family should be called. A warm relationship early may form a helpful bond when death is near. Even if the patient is comatose, he should always be treated with respect, especially in the presence of his loved ones.

After death, the focus of concern belongs with the survivors. An elderly person who has lost a spouse will need emotional support to adjust to the loss, and perhaps practical assistance as well. Family members, because of unresolved guilts or other feelings, may need aid to cope with their grief. Many nurses now follow up with families with phone calls or visits to express their *continuing* concern.[9]

SPECIAL PROBLEMS OF THE HOSPITAL ENVIRONMENT

The hospital environment is centered around saving lives; cure and rehabilitation are the goals. It is no wonder that the dying often find themselves "out of phase" in the hospital. Some studies suggest that both nurses and physicians tend to spend significantly less time with dying patients than with those expected to recover.[8] Dying is simply contradictory to the main thrust of hospital activity. Modern life-saving techniques, such as organ transplants and suction tubes, exemplify the prevailing hospital attitude of science over death.

An intensive care unit (ICU) may be particularly unsuitable for the elderly dying patient.[10] Where heroic life-saving techniques are the business of the day, the patient's wishes are sometimes completely overlooked.

> He may cry for rest, peace and dignity, but he will get infusions, transfusions, a heart machine, or tracheotomy if necessary. He may want one single person to stop for one single minute so that he can ask one simple question—but he will get a dozen people around the clock, all busily preoccupied with his heart rate, pulse, electrocardiogram, or pulmonary functions, his secretions or excretions but not with him as a human being.[2]

Not only are the bodies of dying patients sometimes manipulated without regard to their individuality or their wishes, but the psychic needs of the dying are difficult to satisfy in the ICU atmosphere. When they have great need to communicate with their family and friends, visiting is limited, time is very brief, and conversation is hampered by the strange environment and masses of equipment.

The time is gone when people normally died at home among their loved ones. Now 60–80% of all deaths occur in hospitals or nursing homes.[8] Because of modern medical practices, these deaths are often lingering and isolated. Nurses are in a unique position to alleviate the isolation of the dying patient and to bring comfort and understanding. This is particularly true since physicians often have a difficult time relating to their dying patients.

Physicians and the Dying

Physicians are often extremely reluctant to admit that they have no solution for their dying patients. They usually perceive their role as a healer and a saver of lives and may consider any death a personal failure. For a number of reasons, many doctors hesitate to speak frankly with their patients about death. A physician may feel that his patient will give up all hope, or he may not be able confidently to judge the prognosis of a disease. Doctors know only too well the limits of their art—death may come when it is least expected, and some patients survive who have "no chance" of medical cure. The physician's own strong fears of death and his commitment to saving lives may hinder his communication with a dying patient. A professor of psychiatry has expressed the belief that physicians may have a significantly higher aversion to death than do other people.[11]

Kubler-Ross reports that physicians were extremely reluctant to cooperate with her when she first began her interviews with dying patients in Billings Memorial Hospital in Chicago.[2] They felt unanimously that their patients would be either unwilling or unable to talk. It has also been pointed out that patients often find it easier to talk about their feelings with nurses than with their physicians.[12] One man said that it's difficult to carry on a conversation with his doctor, "since he comes in with a stethoscope in his ears and sticks a thermometer in my mouth."[3]

Of course, these generalizations are not always true. A good many doctors favor frank discussions with their dying patients, usually when they feel the patient is ready to know. Certainly, most doctors are aware of the problem:

> There have been times when I haven't been able to cope with an individual patient in a terminal situation, and in a cowardly way, I have run to the stereotyped role of myself as a scientist and technical expert, who doesn't concern himself with people's feelings.[3]

Furthermore, the attitudes of physicians about death and dying are rapidly changing. A great deal of attention has recently been directed toward the dying patient, and one result is the birth of a new medical subspecialty.

Thanatology

The Foundation of Thanatology, begun in 1967 by four professors at Columbia University College of Physicians and Surgeons, is dedicated to the idea of death with dignity. The group holds regular workshops, publishes three journals and a number of books. The Institute for the Study of Humanistic Medicine in San Francisco is another example of the trend toward personalizing all medical care, including the care of the dying. Health professionals there study ways to improve the nontechnological side of care-giving.

Recently the American Hospital Association issued a 12-point bill affirming the right of the individual to choose death by refusing medical treatment and his right to full information.

All these groups, and several others, wish to remove the dying process and its depersonalizing, mechanical context.

Euthanasia

A further manifestation of our current concern with the dying and another protest against the hospital way of dying is the emergence of lay groups interested in protecting the rights of the dying. The Euthanasia Education Council, which advocates only voluntary, passive, euthanasia, has more than 15,000 members. The Council distributes a "Living Will" (100,000 copies had been requested by 1973) which states, among other things:

> If there is no reasonable expectation of my recovery from physical or mental disability; I request that I be allowed to die and not be kept alive by artificial means or heroic measures.

The demand for copies of the Living Will doubled following the Quinlan case.[13]

The question of euthanasia is especially, though by no means exclusively, relevant to the elderly, since older patients choose to die more often than younger patients. Since the general health of older people is likely to be more vulnerable, the hope for "miraculous cure" is diminished. Health professionals frequently report encounters with older patients who do not choose to live.

Belknap has written about an 83-year-old man, Mr. S.F., with cancer of the prostate.[14] Mr. S.F. was extremely weak, had lost control of his bladder and bowels, and was depressed. A proud and independent man, he was ashamed of his weakness and lack of self-control. Belknap first began an aggressive rehabilitation program. The doctor hoped to restore his patient's self-esteem and his interest in life. Belknap was deeply disappointed when Mr. S.F., after 2 weeks, refused to eat. He had great affection and admiration for S.F., and his own values and hopes were symbolized for him in this patient. Through a process of internal self-examination, he came to understand that S.F. wished to die and was able to support him.

> I attended a dying patient at his bedside over a period of four weeks, . . . and was able to assist him in maintaining his personal integrity and dignity. My awareness of my own feelings and wishes enabled me to acknowledge my patient's wishes as separate and distinct from my own, and to support his decision to die.[14]

Mr. S.F. fasted for 9 days before requesting any food. He then ate a small pudding and drank a little water. He resumed his fast, and died 6 days later.

Two men wrote about their grandfather's death.[15] At 81, the grandfather was suffering from severe confusion and disorientation. He, too, chose to die, and refused food and drink. His family supported him in his decision. They respected their grandfather's right to choose.[15]

It is believed that euthanasia is often practiced, but rarely admitted. Passive euthanasia, by disconnecting life-support systems, is probably the most common form of euthanasia. Physicians who are reluctant to face this responsibility may leave orders for nursing staff. Euthanasia is, at present, illegal.

Roberts refers to several instances in which elderly patients, who wish to die rather than live severely curtailed lives, pull at their suction tubes or pacemaker wires.[11] They struggle to die despite the opposition of the whole hospital organization. Although their numbers are small (most people, young and old, do wish to live), these patients present a distressing dilemma for care-givers. Health professionals are divided about the best possible course of action. The patient's right to a dignified death, the staff's commitment to preserving life, the prognosis of the illness, and the family's feelings all must be considered. Although decisions are made by the physician, nurses often feel compelled to share their knowledge of the patient. Staff cooperation and discussion should underlie the decision-making process.

The Hospice Approach

The most promising alternative to the hospital environment for the care of the dying person, old or young, is the hospice. Very successful in England, hospices are now being organized in the

United States as well: in New Haven, Santa Barbara, and in Marin County, California. Since the American hospices are all still in the early stages of development, the British hospices are still the more useful models for study.

A hospice, designed to provide comfort and support for the dying of any age, avoids the cold, impersonal atmosphere too often found in nursing homes and the focus on cure found in hospitals. At St. Joseph's and St. Christopher's in England—the two hospices most widely known—the atmosphere is homelike and relaxed. Since the hospice staff is not responsible for diagnosis or treatment decisions, they are free to expend all their effort in relief and understanding. Not all hospice patients are near death, but none are well enough for rehabilitation. Hospices do not use heroic measures to prolong life. They have no resuscitation. The hospice is closely coordinated with a home-care program. Patients remain at home for as long as possible, and move back and forth from home to hospice. The hospice is actually a back-up unit for comprehensive home care.

The hospice program emphasizes four points: The first is flexibility; a hospice strives to adapt the plan of care to each individual's particular needs. The second emphasis is on patient involvement in the decision-making process. Patients are encouraged to participate in the planning of their care, as well as in maximizing self-care as much as possible. The third focus is on family involvement. In contrast to the hospital environment, in which the family is often made to feel useless and unwanted, in the hospice the family is encouraged to join fully in the care of the patient. The fourth point concerns comfort. The British hospices are known for their expertise in alleviating pain and other discomforts. Brompton's mixture—a formula containing morphine, alcohol, and chloroform water—is used at St. Christopher's with much success and is being used in the American hospice home-care programs. They believe that pain is controlled more successfully, and alertness safeguarded, by routine medication than by waiting until medication is requested.

Dr. Cicely Saunders, director of St. Christopher's, believes that the dying person needs warmth and compassion as well as good technical care. The atmosphere at St. Christopher's is relaxed and peaceful. Children of the staff members play on the grounds, and a feeling of "family" is the essence of the atmosphere. One patient remarked, "I am perfectly content to be here and have experienced such peace that, at times, it is quite overwhelming. . . ."[3] Patients at St. Christopher's invariably die so quietly that they need not be moved from the rooms they share with three or five others. Dr. Saunders has written:

> I believe that to talk of accepting death when its approach is inevitable is not mere resignation or submission on the part of the patient, nor defeat or neglect on the part of the doctor; for each of them accepting death's coming is the very opposite of doing nothing.[3]

The growing interest in death with dignity in this country will, almost certainly, generate more hospices in the years to come. Though American hospices may be somewhat different from these British models (notably in their use of heroin), they may provide environments in which the dying patient is understood and comforted. The New Haven Hospice is now operating a home-care program, and plans, modeled after St. Christopher's, for a 44-bed terminal care inpatient facility are complete. Other hospice programs now exist at St. Luke's in New York City and at Harrisburg Hospital, and dozens of planning committees across the country are studying the hospice concept.[13] The hospice movement promises that dying will become, again, a personal and family matter.

St. Francis' "Prayer for Healers" (a modified version) is included here at the end, in the hope that it will help nurses to respond with wisdom—as well as knowledge—to a dying person.[1]

> Lord,
>   Make me an instrument of your health
> Where there is sickness,
>   let me bring cure;
> Where there is injury,
>   aid;
> Where there is suffering,
>   ease;
> Where there is death,
>   acceptance and peace.

Grant that I may not:

So much seek to be justified,
  as to console;
to be obeyed,
  as to understand;
to be honored,
  as to love, . . .
for it is in giving ourselves
  that we heal,
it is in listening
  that we comfort,
and in dying
  that we are born to eternal life.

REFERENCES

[1]Kubler-Ross, E.: *Death: The Final Stage of Growth.* Englewood Cliffs, N.J.: Prentice-Hall, 1975.

[2]Kubler-Ross, E.: *On Death and Dying.* New York: Macmillan, 1969.

[3]Hendin, D.: *Death as a Fact of Life.* New York: W.W. Norton, 1973.

[4]Zopf, D.: "The Dying Patient: Meeting His Needs Could be Easier than You Think." *Nursing '75,* 5(3):16.

[5]Davis, B.A.: "Until Death Ensues." *Nurs. Clin. N. Am.* 7:303, 1972.

[6]Ebersole, P.P.: "Developmental Tasks in Late Life." In *Nursing and the Aged.* Edited by I.M. Burnside. New York: McGraw-Hill, pp. 69-80, 1976.

[7]Stafford, P.G., and Golight, B.H.: *LSD: The Problem-Solving Psychedelic.* New York: Award Books, 1967.

[8]Dempsey, D.: "Learning How to Die." *New York Times,* Reprint, 1971.

[9]Rinear, E.R.: "Helping the Survivors of Expected Death." *Nursing '75*, 5(3)60, 1975.

[10]Roberts, S.L.: "To Die or Not to Die: Plight of the Aged Patient in ICU." In *Psycho-Social Nursing Care of the Aged.* Edited by I.M. Burnside. New York: McGraw-Hill, 1973, pp. 96-105.

[11]Lifton, R.J., and Olson, E.: *Living and Dying.* New York: Praeger, 1974, p. 36.

[12]White, L.: Cited in "Facing the Reality of Death." *San Francisco Chronicle,* April 30, 1973, p. 20.

[13]Kron, J.: "Designing a Better Place to Die." *New York,* March 1, 1975, pp. 43-49.

[14]Belknap, R.: "Dr. B. and Mr. S.F. Collaborate on Death." *Harper's Weekly,* 44:10, 1975.

[15]Jury, M., and Jury, D.: "Gramps." *Psychology Today,* 9(9): 57-65, 1975.

[16]Feifel, H. ed.: *The Meaning of Death.* New York: McGraw-Hill, 1959.

SUGGESTED READING

Jaeger, D., and Simmons, L.W.: *The Aged Ill.* New York: Appleton-Century-Crofts, 1970.

III

Restorative Nursing for the Aged

Chapter 8

Restorative Nursing

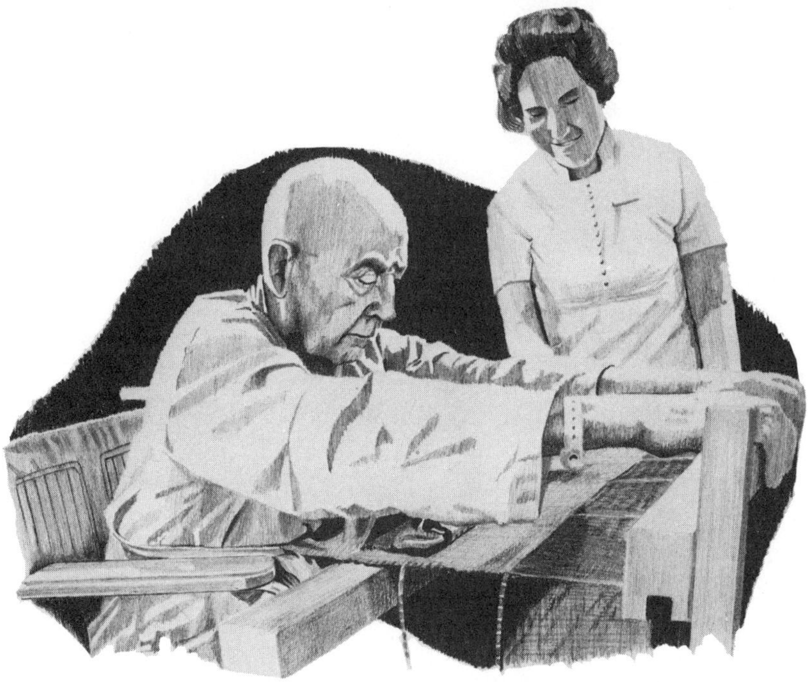

We have discussed the normal physiological and psychosocial processes of aging as well as physical and mental disorders, with some suggested interventions. What is the unifying principle?

Restorative nursing is the key orientation that enables the nurse to care for each patient as an individual to maximize and maintain his level of functioning. It enables her to interact with each patient as fully as possible, utilizing her fund of knowledge and creativity *with* his.

The physical and psychosocial aspects of each person are seen as intrinsically interdependent; neither can operate successfully without the other. Restorative nursing action embraces both.

Restorative nursing is a position of responsibility. It involves continuous decision-making and accountability for those decisions. Nurses need as much knowledge about aging processes as possible, and the cooperation of all the members of the health care team is essential.

Restorative nursing is a willingness to change and find solutions for "insoluble" problems. Every problem is carefully considered and acted upon, not dismissed as impossible. It means that the nurse uses her inventiveness and imagination and enjoys her job.

This chapter, then, is the core of the book. Restorative nursing is the essence of geriatric nursing today.

FUNDAMENTALS OF RESTORATIVE NURSING

Nursing actions vary substantially with each nursing setting. Acute care priorities clearly differ from those of long-term care. Nevertheless, the goal of restorative nursing remains the same: to maximize and protect the functional potential of each patient.

Before specific actions appropriate in each setting are discussed, it is useful to review the fundamentals of restorative nursing, first in terms of goals and assessment, and then in terms of basic care.

Nursing Goals

Restorative nursing begins with diagnosis and continues until the patient achieves his maximum potential. It is not confined to special rehabilitation centers but operates in *all* nursing service. A malfunction or disability may be temporary, permanent, or progressive, and the *general* goal of nursing care depends on which condition is present. In temporary disability, the goal is to return the patient to his former level of functioning. The period of convalescence may be short or long. In permanent disability, the lost function cannot be restored, but the goal is to replace the loss with substitutions (such as prosthetic limbs, special glasses, etc.) whenever possible, and to assist the patient in adjusting to his loss. In progressive disability, in which a function is lost gradually and cannot be replaced by substitution (as in rheumatoid arthritis and Parkinson's disease), the goal is to maintain optimum function for as long as possible while helping the patient adjust to his condition.

Informal rehabilitation is a primary nursing function. Aimed at preventing complications that would retard restoration of lost function, it involves proper bed positioning, frequent turning, meticulous skin care, careful nutrition, and attention to the whole person.[1]

Goals must be individualized in accordance with the unique physical and psychosocial status of each patient. Sometimes an active rehabilitation program entails too much risk and stress for the aged patient. A first step is to make a problem list with the participation of the patient if possible. The chief concerns of such a list are the problems of (1) maintenance or restoration of mobility or activity, (2) maintenance or restoration of contact with reality, and (3) maintenance of social skills and opportunity for meaningful relationship. The nurse must use her knowledge and experience to give proper priority to each problem. Then a nursing care plan can be devised, specifying *what* is to be done, *how, where,* and *by whom.*[2]

Assessment

Assessment means the gathering of information, as an initial step and at any point in the nursing process. Restorative nursing requires both objective and subjective data. Essentially, the nurse needs to determine how much an elderly person wishes someone else to take over some tasks and to what extent the patient can retain control.[3] The participation of the patient is vital to assessment; too often a patient asks for a little help and gets the whole package.

A patient should be assessed in terms of physical and social state, physical and social environment, and in terms of interaction with that environment. How does the patient meet the needs for survival and safety? For love and self-esteem? For meeting the developing requirements of old age, including the prospect of death? Many answers can be found through observation without asking the patient unnecessary (and sometimes embarrassing) questions.[3]

The FANCAP model mentioned in Chapter 4 can be readily used to assess functionality:

Fluids. Does the patient get enough to maintain body function? (High-risk factors include confusion, neurologic deficits that prevent ingestion, depression, and the heavy use of tranquilizers.)

Aeration. Does dyspnea interfere with functional ability? (High-risk factors include congestive heart failure, pulmonary illness, and confinement to bed.)

Nutrition. How does the patient satisfy his nutritional needs? (High-risk factors may be physical or psychosocial. Physical problems include low mobility, neurologic deficits, decubiti, loss of vision or chewing ability, respiratory difficulties, or drug reactions. Psychosocial factors may be poverty, depression, grief, loneliness, or confusion.)

Many older people fall into the high-risk category in reference to nutrition. Any person who regularly eats alone should be suspected of malnutrition and observed for further signs, because eating is so much a social ritual.

Communication. Can the patient give and receive communication sufficiently to meet his physical and social needs? (High-risk factors include aphasia, neurologic deficits, laryngectomy, oversedation. Psychosocial factors may be depression, confusion, a language or cultural barrier, or a crisis state.) Age itself can be a cultural barrier.

Activity. What prevents this person from self-care and mobility?

Pain. Is this person in pain, and does pain interfere with ability to function? (High-risk factors include crisis, oversedation, aphasia, neurologic deficits, and diabetes with neuropathy, in which pain may be a first warning.)[3]

Assessment can lead to insight into perplexing problems:

> Mrs. B. told the nurse she dreaded having her grandchildren visit her. On exploration, the nurse learned that it was not the noise, which the grandmother enjoyed for a short time, or their rowdy affection, which she craved, but the fact that they left the furniture in new positions. Mrs. B. was able to control her environment and live with her decreasing sight as long as no one changed the arrangement of one article in her house, but her knees were black and blue after stumbling into rearranged furniture, and at times, she fell. When she was moved to the hospital for diagnostic work-up, she was panic-stricken and bedbound for she did not know "where anything was."[3]

Each patient's environment should be assessed to determine what factors (architectural features, furniture, lighting, ventilation and heating, kitchen and bathroom equipment, etc.) reduce functional ability, and to discover what can be changed.

Assessment of each patient's functional state, environment, and psychosocial needs is an ongoing process in restorative nursing. It is not only formal and systematic, but also importantly includes subjective judgments and subtle observations—in short, the nurse's feelings. The restorative nurse is *sensitive* and *involved.*

Nursing Activity for Restorative Physical Care

For the patient confined to bed, it is vital to counteract dependency, deterioration, and depression. A rule of thumb is not to do for the patient what he can do for himself.

Proper body positioning, through the use of footboards, sandbags, or pillows, must be maintained to prevent deformities and unnecessary pain. One stroke patient remarked that her paralyzed leg was extremely uncomfortable whenever it lay in an unaligned position.[4]

Frequent turning, every 2 hours, is also essential for the bedridden patient. This, too, is necessary not only for the physical care of the patient but also for his comfort. A stroke patient has written that 1.5 hours is a very long time to wait for a change of position, 2 hours is an eternity, and 2.5 hours a torture.[4]

Maintenance of *range-of-motion* in all joints is a third service to prevent deformities. Range-of-motion exercises may be passive, active assisted (assistance from the nurse), or active (the patient exercises independently). It is necessary to start range-of-motion exercises as soon as it is medically possible, and to know the existing range to avoid pain. Any sign of patient fatigue warrants stopping the exercises. Passive exercises should be repeated three times with each movement to be effective. It is wise to explain to the patient and family that the exercises avoid contractures and muscle atrophy; otherwise, the patient may feel somewhat harrassed.

It is also important to prevent *respiratory complications* in bedridden patients. An immobile patient has a reduced ability to cough, and secretions that accumulate in the lungs may cause hypostatic pneumonia. The nurse conducts daily deep-breathing exercises and encourages deep coughing as part of the routine of restorative care. Frequent turning also helps the patient to expel secretions. Pneumonia is an ever-present threat to bedridden patients, and it is necessary to be alert for elevation in vital signs.

Skin care and the prevention of decubitus ulcers is a fifth need of bedridden patients. A sixth is *adequate nutrition.* There is an increased need for protein to strengthen weakened muscles, and sufficient roughage and fluid (2,000 cc) must be ingested daily for normal excretory functioning. Food high in calcium (milk products, for example) should be minimal for bedridden patients, to avoid renal calculi. Adequate nutrition is sometimes difficult to achieve. Stroke patients may have trouble chewing and swallowing, and almost no one likes to be fed. When a patient is feeding himself, the food tray must be placed carefully, and plenty of time allowed for eating. When he is assisted, eating requires a large measure of time and patience. All mealtime practices should be written and updated on the nursing care plan to insure consistent care.

Finally, *providing for elimination,* whether by bedpan, commode, or other special aids, is another basic nursing service.[1]

Active rehabilitation programs vary with each individual and, to some degree, with different nursing settings. Patients in an acute care center or rehabilitation center usually have a different priority of needs from those of patients in a facility for long-term care.

RESTORATIVE NURSING IN THE HOSPITAL OR REHABILITATION CENTER

Rehabilitation usually involves a health-team approach, including a physician and nurses, often a psychiatrist, a physical therapist, an occupational therapist, a social worker, and sometimes a dietitian and speech therapist as well. The most important person is the patient, who must be interested, enthusiastic, and willing. The nurse has a coordinator role with all the other health team members and is the constant source of support for the patient in the nursing unit.

An initial evaluation to plan an individualized rehabilitation program and to begin discharge planning is the first step in active rehabilitation. The nurse provides essential input for this evaluation and also helps the patient and family participate in the planning process.

One of the early rehabilitative activities is often bladder-and-bowel training. Rehabilitation hospitals usually remove catheters as soon as possible to avoid infection. Bladder training is usually accomplished through a 2-hour toilet schedule and plenty of fluids; bowel training may involve the use of suppositories to establish a regular schedule, though the patient's past habits are often effective stimulants. It is generally not a difficult problem except for patients with severe neurogenic bladder damage.

During rehabilitation, the patient's progress from total dependence toward independence is continually reassessed. All staff should conscientiously support this shift; there is no place for possessiveness or overprotectiveness.

In addition to coordination and support for the patient and family, nursing activity focuses on reteaching self-care, the activities of daily living, and ambulation. The nursing team often must motivate the patient to perform self-care with understanding and firm encouragement. Families can be very helpful by telling the nursing staff about the patient's past interests and by reaffirming staff encouragement.

The procedures for teaching the activities of daily living vary considerably, but some basic rules may apply. It is important to know what the patient has been learning elsewhere to insure continuity of care. Teach simple skills such as hair-brushing and oral hygiene before introducing complex acts such as dressing. Reassurance and positive reinforcement are crucial. It may be helpful to explain procedures fully beforehand and to tackle some problems gradually, step-by-step.

In working with stroke patients, the nurse will find it helpful to remember that damage to the right hemisphere may cause defective reasoning and motor ability without verbal impairment, while damage to the left hemisphere usually affects speech abilities. With patients who have right-hemisphere damage, be on guard against distracting conversation. With patients whose left hemisphere is afflicted, it is necessary to speak slowly and distinctly, and to demonstrate whenever possible. Patients with damage to the right hemisphere often take twice as long to relearn lost skills. They often have impaired comprehension and a short attention span; they may not be able to follow directions, although they may respond appropriately verbally.[5]

The nurse has the additional responsibility to thoroughly instruct the patient and his family about preventive measures. Families should be carefully taught how to prevent pressure sores. In stroke patients, families have to be instructed about safety practices, since the patient may not be able to judge safety adequately.[5]

RESTORATIVE NURSING WITH LONG-TERM PATIENTS

Many patients in long-term facilities have relatively stable disease functions. They are admitted for a host of *other* reasons, such as functional disability (due to physical, mental, or social loss), familial disunity, or simply social displacement. Today many older people cannot be cared for in the community. Although they are admitted by physician's order with a medical treatment plan, other needs are often more important than medical treatment. Even when their medical condition is not stable, other needs may be equally critical.

Yet the medical model dominates long-term care.[6] Medications and medical treatment absorb most of the nurse's time, and little is left for individual assessment. In long-term care, psychosocial problems may be more critical than medical problems. It behooves the nurse to be aware of the patient's *response* to his illness or to aging in general.

Nurses, however, are educated with a medical orientation. As yet, few are taught how to assess and respond to behaviorial problems, especially with reference to older people. Often, when trying to function in this gap, the nurse falls back on custodial care. The medical model dictates primary physical care, and so she gives basic physical care almost exclusively.

There is a need for a restorative nursing model appropriate for long-term care. Many normal nursing responsibilities needed in acute care are out of place in the long-term facility. For example, meticulous input-output records are usually not necessary for bladder-and-bowel training. A "house program" of adequate fluids and roughage and regularly scheduled opportunity to eliminate is often sufficient. The nurse needs a sound background in aging to make her *own* decisions, based on multiple physical and psychosocial factors.

A Nursing Model

In long-term care, the nurse is an independent decision-maker. Nursing is a leadership role. The restorative nursing plan often must be devised with few guidelines from the doctor's admission form.[6]

> A medical description of Mrs. A., with a diagnosis of organic brain syndrome and back osteoarthritis, does not give enough information to plan nursing care. Can Mrs. A. benefit from reality orientation or remotivation? Since it is observed that she depends on sensorimotor activities (walking about, touching, smiling) for stimulation, can she be protected from more severe osteoarthritis? The nursing staff recognizes that if she is confined to bed with no social contact, she will die.[6]

It is the nurse's responsibility to capitalize on the patient's resources and minimize her deficits. The nurse is not a custodian, but rather the therapeutic manager of the patient's care.

Nursing assessment, as mentioned earlier, must include many factors in addition to the medical diagnosis. Some are:

Mobility
Physical strength
Nutritional status
Mental status
Skin
Sensory functions
Speech
Elimination patterns
Daily living activities
Color discrimination
Vital signs
Medications and their possible effects

In long-term care, however, assessment depends on staff observation. It is less quantifiable than in an acute setting. Elaborate assessment forms may be more time-consuming than useful. Care depends on sensitive and informed staff observation and interstaff communication. For this reason, new staff may need a long orientation period.

Summing up long-term care assessment is this notice, found on the wall of the Director of Nursing's office in a convalescent hospital:

NOTICE

The objective of all dedicated company employees should be to thoroughly analyze all situations, anticipate all problems prior to their occurrence, have answers to these problems, and move swiftly to solve these problems when called upon—

However;

When you are up to your ass in alligators, it is difficult to remind yourself that your initial objective was to drain the swamp.

Greenberg has outlined some guidelines for long-term nursing to help the nurse evaluate common changes in a patient's behavior.[6]

1. *Sudden or gradual cessation of food or fluid intake*
A few possible causes are impaction, urinary tract infection, small-stroke syndrome, impending disease processes such as pneumonia or heart failure, or depression. Immediate action is essential. Waiting even a few days to evaluate and intervene may cause irreversible damage to a weakened system. Dehydration, electrolyte imbalance, confusion, and death may result.

2. *Sudden, unexplained falling*
These incidents occur frequently in long-term care facilities. Restorative nursing demands that the *cause* of the fall be assessed, not just its results. Some possible causes, in addition to preexisting neurologic diseases, are transient or permanent heart block or the occurence of paroxysmal cardiac arrhythmia, both causing reduced cerebral blood flow; stroke; undetected audiovisual defects; or psychiatric self-destructive states.

3. *Sudden, irregular slow pulse rate*
Be alert for digitalis toxicity. It is more difficult to detect with confused patients. Any significant behavioral change in a patient on digitalis should signal withdrawing the medication and notifying the doctor.

4. *Sudden or gradual change in sensorium*
Failing vision or hearing may go undetected. It can lead to confusion or falls and sometimes to psychological disorders such as paranoia.

5. *Psychosocial adjustments*
Admission to a long-term facility is a major disruption in any person's life. The patient's past life style, environment, and lifelong coping patterns will influence ability to adjust. It is desirable to make as much leeway as possible for individual life styles, and to respect the patient's needs to collect, hoard, work outdoors, etc. It is also necessary to understand the family's feelings of stress and guilt, and to analyze how these dynamics affect the patient.

It is difficult for anyone to "keep his senses" in a lonely, empty environment. If the medical model is reevaluated, there is *no* need for long-term care facilities to be sterile, empty, impersonal places. In institutions in which restorative nursing is practiced, walls are bright with pictures and color, nurses may not wear uniforms or even use a formal nursing station.

Mirrors and colorful clothing are present everywhere, and the mood is homelike rather than institutional. Patients are not prisoners; they are free to go to school, shop, or take a walk. Families are encouraged to participate in patient care and to take their relatives out whenever possible. Both staff and patients can initiate social activities.

In long-term care, a good recreation program is important. Current events, art lessons, games, and informal gatherings help patients stay in touch with the world and with each other. Often programs such as reality orientation or remotivation are more restorative and rehabilitative than physical therapy.[7] Patient councils can provide a time for expressing dissatisfactions for both patient *and* staff.

Long-term care has its own special problems. A major difficulty at this time is the present state of government regulations. Medicare payments are often inadequate to provide a desirable staff/patient ratio. Facilities that accept only private patients have far more funds with which to operate. Furthermore, government requirements for documentation take more and more valuable time away from direct patient care. In trying to standardize care nationwide, these regulations often burden the *good* programs. Finally, government officials are often more critical than helpful.

Another major problem is the fact of long-term dependency. Patients may wish to live vicariously through the staff; they will love to hear about the nurse's outside activities, her children, etc. The patient may find very few outlets to express independence. Oftentimes, shouting and anger are the only outlets that remain. To encourage self-care, nurses frequently must be firm but never nasty. Nastiness does not work. Perhaps the crucial response to dependency is to maintain respect for the patient. Without such respect, care becomes nontherapeutic.[7]

The long-term caretaker needs special qualities; she must be a warm and patient person. The finest medical care cannot compensate for a lack of these qualities.

THERAPEUTIC TECHNIQUES

The nurse relates to the patient either through a one-to-one relationship or in a group. The question is how to make these relationships therapeutic. This section, in reviewing some rewarding nursing experiences, offers some clues about how to establish and maintain a healing relationship.

The One-to-One Relationship

A one-to-one relationship is achieved through a series of planned, purposeful interactions, in which both the patient and the nurse learn and develop their interpersonal competence. Such a relationship needs closeness and a low level of anxiety. The nurse should be aware of any sensory loss in the patient and communicate appropriately. Touch is an invaluable tool to enhance contact and closeness. To reduce anxiety, watch for fatigue and nonverbal clues. Sharing food often helps to increase closeness. In all relationships, it is indispensable to offer the patient some ray of hope and optimism, for how can a hopeless person relate to anyone?[8]

A public health nurse has described a one-to-one relationship she pursued with an elderly man who was frustrated and angry about his nursing-home situation.[9] She maintained regular, frequent visits, and allowed him to express his anger. She functioned as his advocate with the staff and helped both the staff and patient understand his special needs and keep his anger from accumulating.[9]

Another example of a therapeutic one-to-one relationship involved a nurse with a blind, diabetic, Spanish-speaking elderly woman.[10] The goal of intervention was to alleviate this patient's extreme loneliness, for she was isolated both by physical loss and cultural differences. Through regular visits and ongoing concern, the nurse was able to relieve some of the anxiety and despair that accompanies loneliness.[10]

Groups

The group therapy approach to patient/nurse relationships has diverse applications, from short-term groups for rehabilitating stroke patients (or their families) to long-term groups for severely disoriented patients. Goals vary according to the needs of the groups. Several nurses, some with little or no experience in group leadership, report that groups are a promising structure for many kinds of care.

For long-term institutionalized elderly patients, a group devoted to resocialization, crisis intervention, and a sharing of the life-review process achieved recognizable benefits.[11] The group helped patients, albeit slowly, to become more independent and expand their range of activity. The group leader, working with no previous experience in group therapy, concentrated on introducing new stimuli, helping members meet their own needs, and describing the patients' behavior and appearance to them. She encouraged verbal communication between the patients as well as with her. Family participation was actively promoted.

In another group, organized to provide stimulation and orientation in the back ward of a state hospital, the nurse found that friendship requires no special skills.[12] She notes, however, that a familiarity with gerontology and communication skills is very helpful. Such groups fight "mental bedsores" which develop from the boredom of institutional life.[13] No massive personality reorganization is expected from such groups.

A short-term group for stroke patients in a rehabilitation center may have substantially different goals. Such a group counteracts the physical emphasis of nursing, and makes holistic, personal care a reality. Talking and observing deserve recognition as priority nursing services, and a short-term group is one expression of this awareness. The goal of one such group was to give the patients an opportunity to express their feelings and support one another.[14] The patients talked about their sense of hopelessness and isolation and the depersonalization of the hospital environment. The group served its cathartic purpose and enhanced interaction between patients. It also provided feedback to enrich and direct institutional policies.

SEXUALITY

No discussion of restorative geriatric nursing is complete without reference to sexuality, because sexuality is intrinsic to a person's self-esteem and well-being. The nurse must be able to recognize and accept sexuality in her older patients in order to respond in a therapeutic fashion. To deny the elderly person his sexuality is to deny him identity as a person, and to exercise undue control. This encourages conflict and anxiety in the patient.

Sexual activity in old age is generally regarded as deviant behavior. Perhaps because of the Judeo-Christian emphasis on procreation, our prevailing cultural attitude toward sex in later life is one of hostility. "What is virility at 25 becomes lechery at 65."[15]

This hostility has engendered several myths about old age. Contrary to common belief, sex continues to be important to many old people. Many remain sexually active in their 70s, 80s and even 90s.[16] Sexual activity tends to decrease with advancing age, but the reasons are usually psychological or social rather than physical. The individual may fear social censure or find no available partner or may internalize society's expectations and become psychologically incapable of sexual activity. Male impotence is most often psychogenic in origin, and the majority of inactive women refrain from sex because of marital status.

Physical causes of decreased sexuality are, most commonly, a low level of wellness or a reaction to drugs such as sedatives. As with any individual of any age, all that is necessary is "a healthy body, and a willing partner."

Conflict may arise because the individual does not feel old. Sexuality finds no expression because of society's asexual role expectation. It is important that health professionals not contribute to this conflict.

Another myth of old age is that elderly men are prone to crimes of exhibitionism or child-molesting. This is not substantiated in fact, yet the myth may force people to refrain from normal displays of affection.[16]

> One old man, a resident of a retirement home, used to play with the children on their way home from school. He liked to tease them, and pretend to block their path, and the children apparently enjoyed him. One mother, who thought his behavior was seductive, called the police.[15]

Implications

Much can be done to challenge these attitudes. Health workers need to accept sexuality and refrain from considering it regressive or abnormal. Opportunities for sexuality can be made available in long-term care facilities. Sex counseling before hospital discharge is often indicated to relieve anxiety for patients with gynecologic or prostatic conditions, for cancer patients, and for patients with restricted mobility. Individual sex counseling or marital counseling is often helpful for patients with impotency problems. Hypochondriasis in older women may be related to sexuality and may be amenable to counseling as well.

In conclusion, the stifling of sexuality in older people often leads to the repression of normal displays of affection. Touching is an extremely important way to maintain contact with reality and relieve anxiety. Restorative nursing uses touch *liberally* and accepts touching between patients.

REFERENCES

[1]Birchenall, J., and Streight, M.E.: *Care of the Older Adult.* Philadelphia: Lippincott, 1973.

[2]Wolanin, M.O.: "Nursing Evaluation and Goals." In *Nursing and the Aged.* Edited by I.M. Burnside. New York: McGraw-Hill, 1976, pp. 431–435.

[3]Wolanin, M.O.: "Nursing Assessment." In *Nursing and the Aged.* Edited by I.M. Burnside. New York: McGraw-Hill, 1976, pp. 398–420.

[4]McNeil, F.: Stroke! Nursing insights from a stroke-nurse victim. *RN,* Sept. 1975, pp. 75–81.

[5]Conlon, K.: Kentfield Rehabilitation Hospital, Kentfield, Calif. Interview, Mar. 26, 1976.

[6]Greenberg, B.M., and Zaranka, J.D.: Medical model—nursing model? A gerontological dilemma. *J. Gerontol. Nurs.* 1(4): 6-13, Sept.-Oct., 1975.

[7]Thomas, M.: Marin Convalescent Hospital, Tiburon, Calif. Interview, Mar. 24, 1976.

[8]Burnside, I.M., ed. "One-to-one Relationship Therapy with the Aged." In *Nursing and the Aged.* New York: McGraw-Hill, 1976, pp. 126–135.

[9]Robinson, L.D.: "You Don't Seem to Want to Understand: A Case History." In *Nursing and the Aged.* Edited by I.M. Burnside. New York: McGraw-Hill, 1976, pp. 34–43.

[10]Abarca, M.C.: "One-to-one Relationship Therapy: A Case Study." In *Psycho-Social Nursing Care of the Aged.* Edited by I.M. Burnside. New York: McGraw-Hill, 1973, pp. 25–33.

[11]Blake, D.R.: "Group Work with Institutionalized Elderly." In *Psycho-Social Nursing Care of the Aged.* Edited by I.M. Burnside. New York: McGraw-Hill, 1973, pp. 153–160.

[12]Strange, A.Z. "Around the Kitchen Table: Group Work on a Back Ward." In *Psycho-Social Nursing Care of the Aged.* Edited by I.M. Burnside. New York: McGraw-Hill, 1973, pp. 174–186.

[13]Burnside, I.M., ed. "Long-term Group Work with Hospitalized Aged." In *Psycho-Social Nursing Care and the Aged.* New York: McGraw-Hill, 1973, pp. 202–213.

[14]Holtzen, V.L. "Short-term Group Work in a Rehabilitation Hospital." In *Psycho-Social Nursing Care of the Aged.* Edited by I.M. Burnside. New York: McGraw-Hill, 1973, pp. 161–173.

[15]Burnside, I.M., ed. "Sexuality and the Aged." In *Nursing for the Aged.* New York: McGraw-Hill, 1976, pp. 452–464.

[16]Anderson, Catherin J.: Sexuality in the aged. *J. Gerontol. Nurs.* 1(5): 6–11, Nov.–Dec. 1975.

Much of the information in this chapter was obtained in interviews. We especially thank Charlotte Offhaus, Administrator, Medical Manors, Vallejo, California for her interview on January 25, 1976, and Dolores Tyberg, R.N., San Rafael, California for her interview December 11, 1975.

SUGGESTED READING

Guidelines to Stroke-Patient care. *R.N.* Sept. 1975, pp. 83–84.

Chapter 9

Continuity of Care

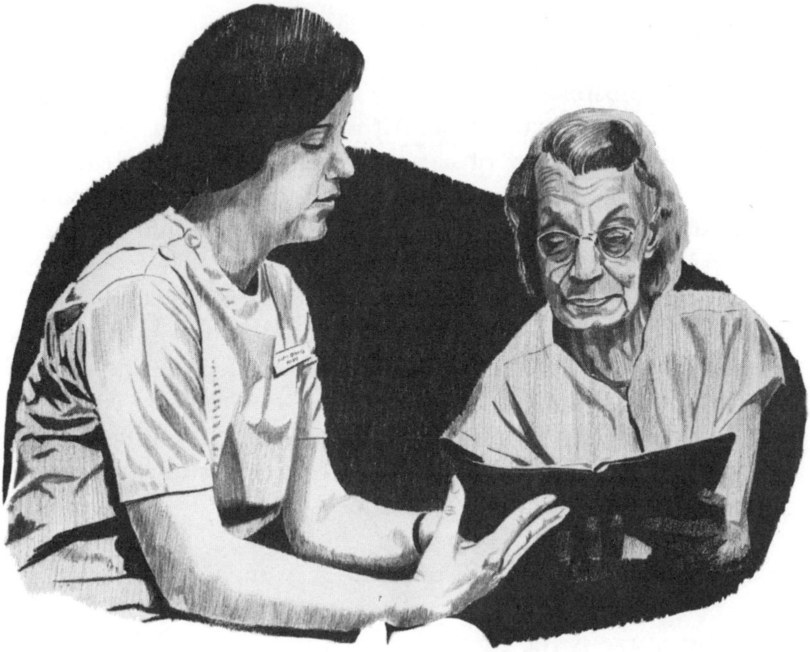

Because illness is often surrounded by a number of related problems, it brings with it a period of transition for the patient and his family. Continuity of care facilitates this transition and protects the patient and his family from unnecessary anguish. Continuing care means that the patient receives uninterrupted care until he reaches his optimal health and rehabilitation potential, and that he is helped to arrange his living circumstances to maintain his health after discharge.

Continuity of care must be maintained from shift to shift, from one hospital service to another, and from the hospital to another facility or to home. Although the focus is on discharge planning, continuity of care in practice involves dealing with the many problems surrounding illness. It is a flexible and integrating function—"creating something when you see the need."[1]

Discharge planning is often crucial to the care of older people. It is indispensable for disabled or chronically ill persons who require long-term care. Persons with amputations, diabetes, emphysema, or stroke, or those who need complicated medications, will need careful planning to guarantee continuity of care. Cancer patients usually require home care service as well. "No one should have to cope with a first colostomy irrigation at home alone."[2] A person whose home environment is not suitable for his care will need help in making better arrangements.

The nurse is the primary initiator in formalizing discharge planning. She knows the patient's capacities and limitations, and can evaluate what he needs. Moreover, she is in the coordinator role, a liaison between the patient, family, and doctor. She is the patient's advocate. In many hospitals today, one person is formally designated to be responsible for continuity of care, and this is, by far, the best arrangement. However, when no one person is responsible, the nurse should fill the gap.

"Every nurse must ask herself who will fill that role if she and her colleagues decline—deliberately or by default."[3]

The Steering Committee of the National League of Nurses Division of Nursing Services strongly recommends that every hospital and nursing home appoint one person, preferably full-time, to develop plans for continuing care and to coordinate a system of referral. Realizing that "what's everybody's business is nobody's business," they urge

> that an all-out effort toward achieving continuity of nursing service be made and emphasize the importance of an *organized referral system,* of a *formally appointed person* to work on continuity of nursing care, and of the need to provide the person in this job with *authority* and *responsibility* to keep the staff aware of patients' continuing nursing needs and to take appropriate action to see that they are met.[4]

Where no continuity-of-care coordinator or liaison nurse is available, the head nurse must accept responsibility for thorough planning, with the cooperation of all staff to provide her with the necessary information. *Someone* must take the initiative to coordinate planning immediately after a patient's admission. The uselessness of excellent acute care when the patient is discharged without appropriate follow-up is clear: Many repeated hospital admissions attest to this need.

Utilization review boards, required in some form in all settings, are coordinated with continuity-of-care programs. The boards determine whether the utilization of beds is proper and conforms to Medicare requirements, and their decisions are incorporated in the planning process. In many cases, their determination is critical, since Medicare provides only for patients who require skilled nursing.

THE FUNDAMENTALS OF CONTINUITY OF CARE

Before the operational elements of continuing care are discussed in detail, it is useful to clarify the basic functions of a continuity of care program. These are:

1. Admissions review. A daily review of admissions forms offers clues about who may have special problems for discharge planning, and provides a good deal of helpful information at the outset.
2. Assessment. Assessment is, of course, the preliminary step for evaluating the patient's needs. Consideration of the patient's needs outside the hospital should start early.

3. Staff coordination and orientation. All staff must be alerted to the patient's need for continuing care, and their input has to be coordinated.
4. Initiating contact. It is best to make contact with the patient and his family early so that a working relationship exists to handle crises or discharge problems.
5. Crisis intervention. Crisis intervention is a large part of a continuity-of-care program. The nurse-coordinator is called upon to help the patient and family cope with drastic changes.
6. Coordination of home evaluation when needed. In some cases, it is necessary to visit the patient's home and to suggest changes to make it a more suitable environment. The planner must see that this is done, and input from the home visit must be integrated into the discharge planning.
7. Patient teaching. The continuity-of-care planner sees that the patient receives careful, unhurried instruction about his home health care. The family may need instruction as well.
8. Liaison with community resources. The continuity-of-care program facilitates the connection between the patient and whatever community resources are appropriate. It protects the patient from becoming lost in endless bureaucracy.
9. Planning post-hospital care. The culmination of discharge planning is the formulation of a comprehensive, practical plan to meet the needs of each patient.
10. A systemized referral procedure. The coordinator organizes a referral system to guarantee that all interfacility referral forms are complete.

In every nursing setting, these ten functions must be integrated in the continuity-of-care program. A description of an excellent continuity-of-care program in terms of these functions will serve to clarify the practical components of continuing care. Guidelines can be drawn from this program, and applied in less ideal settings.

A MODEL CONTINUITY-OF-CARE PROGRAM IN OPERATION

Marin General Hospital is a medium-sized acute hospital in Marin County, Calif. Located close to San Francisco, it has access to a great many community resources available only in metropolitan areas. The hospital's continuity-of-care program is staffed full-time by Nurse-Director Faith Bartlett, a social worker, and a secretary.

Admissions Review

The continuity-of-care office receives a copy of every admission form. Each new patient is evaluated for potential problems; a good deal of useful information can be easily gleaned from these forms. (For example, these forms will show the patient's age, admission diagnosis, chronic conditions, financial circumstances, whether he has close family, etc.)

No doctor's orders are necessary to initiate contact with the patient, although doctors frequently refer family members to the continuity-of-care office soon after admission. Physicians may not consider discharge planning until after the acute condition is stabilized. Therefore, the program operates independently to provide early contact, using the admissions information to judge—on a preliminary basis—which patients are potential clients.

Early contact with the patient and his family is desirable on three counts: (1) It allows time to do thorough assessment and instruction. (2) It helps to establish a rapport that may be invaluable at a later date. (3) Whenever medically possible, the patient's participation in the planning process contributes *directly* to his improvement.[3]

Assessment

Once contact is made, the process of assessment begins. Conferences with nursing staff, and an evaluation of the information gained from nursing assessment interviews, provide input for planning. The office has organized conferences with *all* nursing staff in three units (the orthopedic, radiotherapy, and physical therapy units) on a weekly basis. These free-ranging discussions provide information to the continuity-of-care office, coordinate assessment, and allocate responsibilities (such as patient instruction, etc.) to specific people, and give nurses and aides someone to whom to bring their concerns and problems. The director is also accessible in an informal way because she visits the wards each day. Staff cooperation and concern is absolutely essential to the operation of the program.

Staff Coordination

Bartlett has some important suggestions to make in reference to staff-program coordination.[1] First, she explains the continuity-of-care program and purpose to each new staff member during the first week of orientation. In this particular institution, it has been found desirable to do this on Friday, since by that time new personnel are acquainted with some patients and already actively concerned about their future care.

Secondly, she relies on the nursing assessment form for valuable input and works to help nurses use this tool in a constructive way. These interviews with patients should not be rushed or mechanical. If it takes a day or two for the nurse to find time to converse in a relaxed fashion with each new patient, this is preferable, by far, than a hurried interview. The patient himself may need a little time to accommodate himself to the hospital environment and feel willing to answer more questions.

To clarify her own thoughts and to use as a teaching tool, Bartlett has outlined a nursing assessment format that covers the essential points of concern for planning.[1] The format is reprinted here to aid nurses in checking their own assessments.

> In planning with the patient and his family for his return to the community, it is necessary to have the following information:
>
> A. Information from front sheet re: name, age, admission diagnosis, etc.
>
> B. Health status:
>
> 1. Independence and self-care ability
> 2. Orientation, degree of mental alertness, cooperation
> 3. Elimination problems, incontinence, catheters

4. Speech, hearing, vision impairment
5. Motor ability

C. Home situation, family make-up, occupation:
1. If patient lives alone, are there family/friends to help?
2. If ambulation impaired, is house on one level, bathroom near bedroom, apartment on first floor, etc.?
3. Is patient retired, wage-earner? When can he return to job?

D. Equipment, medications, diet, therapy:
1. Assistive devices as necessary, i.e., wheelchair, walker, intermittent positive-pressure breathing.
2. Medications?
3. Special diet for family/patient to learn. (Always good to have conference with dietitian *before* day of discharge, including sample menus for patient to take home.)
4. Is physical therapy, occupational therapy, speech therapy, or inhalation therapy to be continued after discharge?

E. Financial
1. Is hospital covered by private insurance, Medicare, Medi-Cal, County?
2. Is there need for financial aid and counseling?

F. Approximate length of stay, and doctor's plan for post-hospital care.

Early Contact

It is necessary to make early contact with the patient and his family, and to coordinate the interaction of the various members of the health team long before discharge. It takes time for nurses, physicians, physical therapists, dietitians, occupational therapists, and social workers to share ideas and integrate activities. The patient has the right to exercise control over the planning process, and it is important to talk to the family as soon as possible. Their feelings and needs should be understood and incorporated in planning. (For example, one family may feel that they can no longer cope with the care of an aged, ill relative; another may strongly desire their relative to return home.) *Every situation is different,* and it takes time to establish a working relationship.

Crisis Intervention

A large part of the work of this continuity-of-care program involves crisis intervention. Illness or accidents frequently precipitate a crisis for the patient and/or his family. The nurse and social worker are called upon to intervene with timely support, creative problem-solving methods, and the encouragement of new coping mechanisms.

A family may struggle to maintain an aged relative in their home despite overwhelming obstacles. They may find planning for alternative care extremely upsetting. A patient may become distraught about his illness or the possibility of relocation. The continuity-of-care office assumes the ongoing responsibility of intervening whenever possible.

Home Evaluation

The program arranges for home visits by public health nurses or others whenever it seems necessary. Home evaluations are particularly important for patients with long-term disabilities. A visit may ascertain whether the home layout is adequate (bath downstairs, access to outdoors, etc.) and check the need for special equipment such as grab bars, ramps, and kitchen and bathroom equipment. Local rehabilitation centers are often good sources of suggestions about how to build whatever is needed.

If a home situation seems inadequate, the patient may be referred to the appropriate community agency for assistance in locating a more suitable home. Bartlett emphasizes that the patient has a right to be in control.[1] Nurses can offer alternatives, but the choice belongs to the patient.

Occasionally it is helpful for the patient to return home for a brief trial period before discharge. This may help to pinpoint problem areas and suggest solutions.

Patient Teaching

The continuity-of-care office is responsible for coordinating patient teaching, seeing to it that the necessary instruction is done, and that enough time is allocated for careful teaching. Haphazard patient teaching can lead to complications and severe set-backs. Sometimes, follow-up instruction by public health nurses or home nursing personnel is also indicated.

Patient teaching should be carried on with the patient's home environment in mind. For example, a colostomy patient will need to schedule at-home irrigations for a time when the bathroom will be available. It is best for a nurse to ascertain this kind of information early to avoid initiating an inappropriate schedule.

If a patient has special dietary requirements, it is often helpful if the dietitian talks with the patient, determines his special likes and dislikes, and devises an individualized suggested menu. Older people often have difficulty changing long-established eating habits, and may need specific guidelines to avoid malnutrition. Lists of do's and don'ts may not suffice.

Liaison with Community Resources

In Marin County, Calif., the role of liaison with community resources is a complex one. The area is resource-rich, and many rural localities do not have comparable circumstances. Perhaps the chief resource for almost all places is the *public health department.* A public health nurse can do indispensable follow-up care if the patient is receptive. This nurse can respond to any problems that develop after discharge. Home nursing agencies may also perform this function, but Medicare usually does not cover this service.

Public health departments can be encouraged to extend their service to senior citizens if needed. For example, the Marin County department has a full-time geriatric consultant who is highly skilled in the care of older people and teaches in convalescent hospitals in addition to other nursing functions.

Convalescent hospitals, rehabilitation centers, and *nursing homes* are another major resource. Bartlett has visited all the facilities in her area, and continually evaluates the care they provide in order to make knowledgeable referrals.[1] She feels that family feedback is usually a reliable indicator of the quality of care. In deciding which facility to recommend, the planner must consider many factors. The chief determinants are the quality of care available, the special needs of the patient, and a location near the family and the doctor.

Boarding houses are also available in many areas, and offer some supportive care in an independent and sociable environment. They are another important resource for older people.

Senior citizen groups also provide needed service. As in Marin, they may have a Meals on Wheels program to serve hot food to housebound people; they may meet transportation needs; they often publish newsletters with information about legislative developments, financial and legal aid, and social events. In Marin County, the senior citizen groups are extremely active and effective. It may be helpful to refer patients or their families to local groups as well as to review their newsletters.

The *American Cancer Society,* the *American Heart Society,* and the *Diabetes Association* are useful resources. For example, the American Cancer Society often offers low-cost home equipment, transportation, and individual and group counseling to cancer patients. *Local rehabilitation centers* may have special groups as well. One in Marin County has a group for families of stroke patients.

Home health services provided by visiting nurse associations or home nursing agencies are often needed by older patients. They usually offer more extensive care than the public health department can provide, but they may prove too costly for some patients.

Social service agencies, either public or private, are instrumental in the care of people with financial or social problems. County-administered social service departments may have special programs for blind or disabled persons or homemaking services in addition to providing financial relief. Religious charitable organizations (Catholic welfare bureaus, Jewish welfare organizations, or Protestant welfare organizations) can be contacted through the churches and synagogues; they offer social services and sometimes financial aid.

Bartlett has tapped another unusual community resource: *Nursing students* at a near-by college (registered nurses who are working for baccalaureate degrees) need clinical experience and are often glad to visit patients at home and assess their care.[1]

Each community may have unique resources as well. Outstanding individuals may be involved in relevant community work, and contact with such people is sometimes invaluable. In

Marin County, one older, disabled man is dedicated to helping other disabled persons and has organized an Indoor Sports Group.

Each locality needs to compile its own list of available community resources. Near-by continuity-of-care specialists may be tapped for information. This list—essential for any continuity-of-care program—should be placed on every patient care unit where the information can be disseminated to all nurses. Bartlett has drawn up a problem-resource sheet for her locale, complete with phone numbers (Table 9.1). It should be remembered that the patient must be receptive before any community resource can be activated.

Discharge Plan

The continuity-of-care office prepares a post-hospital-care plan with the cooperation of all the members of the health team. The plan encompasses the patient's health status (self-care ability, orientation, communicative ability, locomotion, etc.), his home and family situation, his need for special equipment, medications, or diet, and his financial status. The plan *specifically* indicates the source of needed equipment, home changes, and instruction.

A Referral System

Finally, the office supervises the preparation of a complete, up-to-date interfacility referral form whenever needed. These forms are especially important in extended-care settings, for they communicate information about established patterns, likes and dislikes, etc.

A schedule of the current activities of the continuity-of-care program is a good way to summarize these diverse functions.

On a daily basis, the continuity-of-care office staff

- Make rounds to each nursing unit to assess needs of new patients, visit patients, are available for problems, and obtain information regarding progress
- Have individual conferences with patients and families
- Phone referrals

Supervise the preparation of interfacility forms
Update patients' records
Do problem-solving
Interpret Medicare regulations

On a weekly basis, they
Sit down with each head nurse and review plans for all patients
Have conferences with physiotherapy, radiotherapy, and orthopedic units
Visit community resources
Confer with the director of nursing
Attend the nursing service council

On a monthly basis, they
Attend committe meetings and regional meetings.

Other activities include introducing the program to various disciplines, attending team conferences and hospital education programs, visiting other facilities, and coordinating field trips for other nurses.

Table 9.1. Problem-Resource Sheet

Need	Community resources
Attendant care; homemaker; private duty nursing	Agencies furnishing nursing or homemaker services
Visiting nurse	Public health nurse or nursing services
Equipment	Rental companies; medical supply companies; American Cancer Society
Transportation	Ambulance service; American Cancer Society; senior citizen groups
Housing	Local police department; emergency housing organization
Financial problems	Department of social services
Special visitors	Ostomy club; mastectomy club
Other useful numbers	Suicide prevention contacts; community switchboard; etc.

Discharge Planning for Long-term Patients

Continuity of care is relevant not only to acute hospital settings. A different kind of program involving long-term patients in a veteran's hospital has been described by Conti.[5]

Discharge planning was initiated for patients who had been institutionalized for several years. These people were usually very dependent due to their long hospitalization. Yet the program was successful in relocating many patients to other care settings and thereby restoring them to a fuller level of functionality.

Planning was done only with the consent of the patient and with his participation. It was in no way authoritarian. The long-term patient needs continuous staff support to cope with relocation. Staff members also may need help to break ties with long-term patients. The program initiated prerelease groups to discuss the problems of relocation and provide counseling service. Families were involved whenever possible.

An essential component of this program was extensive follow-up. All patients were visited after release at least once a month by a staff member, and usually much more often. Staff members consulted with new care-givers, and explained each patient's unique needs. For example, one patient characteristically wore his pajamas under his clothing all day and put on fresh pajamas at night. The staff worked to protect his right to continue his unusual, but in no way harmful, personal habits.

Staff and patients, both those who were released and many who remained, were encouraged and invigorated by this program. The new initiative to return long-term patients to the community significantly improved morale and stimulated new ways of thinking about each patient's capacities.

Special Problems of Continuing Care

Costs are often a serious problem in planning continuity of care. Medicare does not cover supportive nursing; it is limited to acute hospitals and skilled nursing facilities. Very often, elderly patients require only supportive nursing after they are discharged from the acute hospital. Moreover, many private health-insurance plans have similar limitations.

This problem, a very real one, highlighting a terrible gap in national health-care service, is often compounded by emotional connotations. It may be difficult for the patient or his family to cope with the connection between needed care and costs. Misinformation about insurance plans may lead to much frustration and confusion. The alternative—social-welfare agencies' covering the costs of supportive nursing when the patient is unable to pay—is often emotionally upsetting to the individual and his family. Moreover, social-welfare agencies usually do not assume costs until virtually all the patient's own resources are spent.

The coordinator works to devise a plan that meets both the medical needs and the financial capacities of the patient and helps the patient and family accept some unavoidable compromises. Some older people are extremely reluctant to accept financial relief and may need careful explanations.

Another common problem arises when the patient is unwilling to accept the suggestions of health personnel. He has the right to evaluate the alternatives available and control his own planning. In fact, patient participation in the planning process is a major therapeutic step. When a patient insists on going home to an inadequate environment and is unwilling to accept available home assistance, and especially when it seems that he is going home to die, the care-giver is in a frustrating position. The challenge is to find a creative solution that is acceptable to the patient; sometimes this is not possible.

What can be done in a situation where *no one* can take responsibility for coordinating continuing care? A partial solution may be found in rigorous systematization. A fixed schedule for review of discharge planning should be established, pinpointing needs and utilizing all the resources of the health team. The nursing care plan should incorporate discharge considerations, include notes about family conferences, and be kept current. In a small hospital setting, these efforts may significantly help to provide continuing, uninterrupted care for all patients.

REFERENCES

[1]Bartlett, F.: Interview, Jan. 13, 1976. Marin General Hospital.

[2]Birchenall J., and Streight, M.E.: *Care of the Older Adult.* Philadelphia: Lippincott, 1973.

[3]David, J.H., Hanser, J.E., and Madden, B.W.: "Guidelines for Discharge Planning." Rancho Las Amigas Hospital, Inc., Downey, Calif., 1968.

[4]National League of Nursing: "Statement of Continuity of Nursing Care." The Steering Committee of the National League of Nurses, Division of Nursing Services, New York, 1966.

[5]Conti, M.L.: "Continuity of Care for Elderly Discharged Hospital Patients." In *Psycho-Social Nursing of the Aged.* Edited by I.M. Burnside. New York: McGraw-Hill, 1973, pp. 100–121.

Chapter 10

What's New?

Somehow or other the whole world is my new world. It's new in the sense of energy, of producing, of meeting friends on a new level. . . . I do honestly feel cosmic.

—Eleanor Karbach, 73[1]

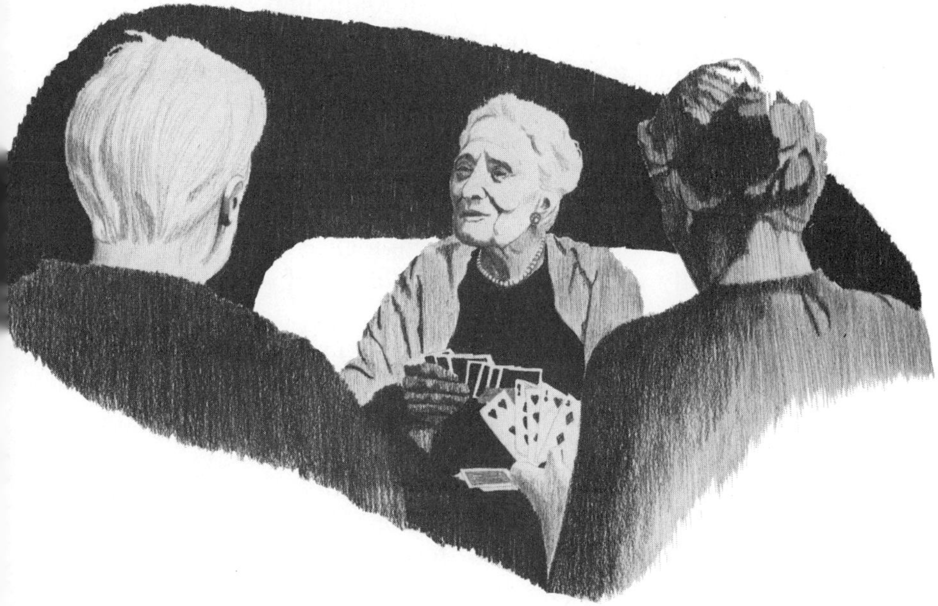

It *is* a whole new world for many older people today, and a new world for the helping professions as well. Basic attitudes about old age are changing; expectations are being transformed; newly acquired knowledge is being assimilated and applied. A fundamental shift in the orientation of geriatric nursing has occurred in recent years—a shift away from custodial care to holistic restorative nursing. Simultaneously, a shift in the attitudes of people, both old and young, about the potentialities of old age is taking place. The old are learning to expect more in their later years; senior citizen groups of many kinds are springing up. Together, these changes create a strikingly new environment for geriatric nursing.

There remains a big difference of course, between the ideal and the available care being offered for older people. These changes in geriatric nursing are fundamental ones, and progressive, up-to-date geriatric care is not yet common. It is often necessary to make the best of existing circumstances while keeping sights set on improvements in the direction of enlightened care.

In the realm of physical care, dramatic progress has been made in the treatment of diseases common to old age, such as cancer and atherosclerosis. In psychological care, the potential for reversibility in functional disorders and acute brain syndrome has been amply demonstrated.

In general, *it is now recognized that (1) prevention, (2) thorough evaluation, and (3) genuine therapeutic efforts are essential to the care of the old.* The therapeutic goal for each individual requires careful determination.

In some cases, maintenance of a patient's condition is a challenging goal in itself; it may require great effort and afford much satisfaction. This kind of maintenance is quite different from custodial care. Curative nursing, so sadly neglected in the past with respect to older people, is now recognized as a primary function.

The patient with chronic organic brain syndrome is no longer cared for only by changing the bedpans, bedclothes, and position. Now nurses are finding that care includes conversation, touch, reality orientation, behavior modification, and a physical exam. They are also finding that the patient responds positively to this kind of therapy.

An elderly stroke victim was often considered nontreatable in the past. Now a careful evaluation of his disability is made and appropriate physical and speech therapies are initiated as soon as possible.

Education

The three functions of nursing demand awareness of the new developments in gerontology and flexibility and innovation as new techniques are introduced. Unfortunately, preparation for geriatric care has not "caught up" with these changes. Very few schools offer special programs in geriatrics, and the care of older people is neglected in the basic education of most nurses. The information needed for competent care of the old is not readily available, and must be actively sought out by individual nurses.

Several schools across the country do offer comprehensive programs in geriatric nursing on the graduate level. Among these are Case Western Reserve University, Texas Women's University, Duke University, and the Universities of Arizona and Colorado. Other nursing schools offer some graduate courses in gerontology. The lack of special attention to geriatrics in schools of nursing and in medicine on the undergraduate level (there is now no chair of Gerontology anywhere in the United States) reflects the old attitudes of neglect and disinterest. As the field attracts more and more attention and concern, we can expect the schools to respond with more adequate programs. Geriatrics may well become part of the core curriculum of nursing education in the not-too-distant future.

New developments in geriatrics are occurring on three crucial levels: (1) in attitude, (2) in knowledge, and (3) in the economic circumstances of the aging person and the consequent availability of medical care.

THE NEW ATTITUDE

Now we see the old as people. Cultural attitudes in the past have blinded medical professionals to the potentials of old age. Recent work has established the value of restorative care and liberated us from the old cultural mythology. Old people are responsive to therapy; many of their ailments are reversible. Just as it is for people of all ages, treatment *is* worth while.

Many nurses are discovering that working with older people, especially in a restorative environment, is both fun and satisfying.

Tyberg, a director of nursing who worked in a convalescent hospital in which restorative nursing approaches are used, said, "I'd walk in at seven o'clock. It was just *joy!* 'Good morning, Dolores! Good moorrning, Doloores!' (That's Joe.)"[2]

The old attitudes, however, persist and are difficult to shake. Recently a nurse in another convalescent hospital said, "There is no solution to old age."

The essence of the new attitude is just the opposite: There may be no solution to old age, but there definitely are solutions to the problems of old age.

There is, in fact, a range of solutions, of approaches that require tailoring to meet individual needs. In many cases, the techniques are not new; only their application to older people is new. Even elementary techniques of care and counseling often meet with great success because, for so long, nothing was attempted with older patients. Particularly important is the comprehensive evaluation of each individual, since conditions in the aged oftentimes go long unrecognized.

The key to the "solution" to old age is in our attitude toward it and, ultimately, in the attitudes of the old themselves. As Beauvoir wrote: "The only solution to the problems of old age is for each old person to go on pursuing ends that give existence a meaning."[3]

How can we support and encourage this pursuit?

THE NEW KNOWLEDGE

We have seen that a holistic approach to health care, with a recognition of the interplay of many and varied forces, underlies modern gerontologic thought. It is useful to summarize now some of the other basic concepts that have been discussed earlier in this book; these notions are the fundamentals of the new knowledge in the field.

Multiple-systems interaction. In geriatrics, the emphasis on multiple-systems interaction is especially strong. Because the systems of many older people function near peak tolerance level, stress on any one system often affects others. The care of older patients therefore requires special attention to the interaction of multiple factors. As drug tolerances are usually lower, the pharmaceutical treatment of one condition often triggers another. Physical ailments often present themselves as mental confusion in older patients. Psychic stress more readily leads to somatic symptoms. The interaction of multiple factors is, therefore, of critical importance.[4]

The importance of stress. Research indicates that tolerance to stress decreases in old age, whereas the incidence of stress usually increases. Dramatic life change, such as retirement, widowhood, or moving is common in old age; these sources of distress contribute directly to both physical and mental disease.

Old age is often (perhaps always) accompanied by social stress; changes in income, status, or social contact are inevitable. Social stress is responsible for much mental and physical deterioration; therefore, social needs are also important with the elderly.

Marked individual differences. Repeatedly in gerontological literature, researchers emphasize extreme individual differences among the elderly. Preconceived assumptions have no place in geriatric care.

Positive holistic therapy. The elderly are very responsive to a supportive environment (no doubt because they often lack one). Since the medical profession has the greatest access to the elderly population, it is our responsibility to supply holistic help. Rehabilitation is linked to the patient's self-concept and his personal motivation; therapy needs to be directed toward both the psyche and the soma of the person. Current therapies are aggressive and positively oriented. Success is expected and pursued.

Successful old age. Underlying positive therapy is the notion of old age as a challenging and satisfying time of life. Old age is seen within the context of the entire life cycle, with particular developmental tasks to accomplish.

Continuity of care. Comprehensive discharge planning is especially relevant to the needs of the elderly. Discharge planning involves working with the patients and their families, on an individual basis, and finding suitable, supportive environments for people who require extended care. In many areas, discharge planning is confronted with grave difficulties as adequate facilities are often not available. Because of the importance of such planning in geriatric care, Chapter 9 is devoted to this subject.

New opportunities for the elderly are arising, born of our new attitudes about old age. One interesting example in Berkeley, California, is SAGE (Senior Actualization and Growth Explorations). Organized in 1974 by a psychotherapist, Gay Luce, with the help of a family counselor and a therapist with extensive experience in body therapies and Gestalt psychology, SAGE uses a number of techniques to alter negative attitudes about aging and to help people enjoy a rich, creative old age. Their methods include dance, music, massage, deep breathing, and biofeedback, among many others. They try any technique appropriate to the revitalization of body and mind. So far, the group has met with highly gratifying success. Participants report that they feel better than they've *ever* felt. Dr. Harold Wise of Montefiore Hospital, New York City, calls SAGE "the most significant advance in health care in the last 20 years."

One implication of the work done by SAGE (among others) is that many community resources commonly reserved for the young would be helpful to the elderly as well. Many communities have yoga classes, T'ai Chi classes, massage classes, and dance classes, for example, from which everyone might benefit. Special classes of this kind for the elderly might also be useful, in the SAGE spirit.

THE NEW ECONOMICS

Elderly people who live on fixed, limited incomes, often cannot afford the high costs of medical care. Since the enactment of

Medicare and Medicaid legislation in 1965, government financing has made health care much more accessible to many older people. At the same time, because of intricate government regulations and bureaucracy, the *kind* of health care available to the elderly is often less than ideal. The quality of care available to the elderly is determined, in large measure, by political circumstances and changeable government spending priorities.

Medicare is not all-inclusive. It now covers approximately 43% of the average elderly person's health expenses.[5] At this time, it does pay for a large portion of hospitalization and of many outpatient and home health services, doctor bills, and medical supplies. It does not now include coverage for dentures, eyeglasses, outpatient drugs, or physical examinations outside the hospital. These excluded items are, unfortunately, all of special importance to the elderly. The legislators, in trying to restrict excessive use of the program, devised regulations that in some cases, encourage increased spending. Hospitalization is required for a physical exam; the elderly cannot afford preventive care, and conditions are often not treated until they become acute.

Medicare coverage for psychiatric care is unrealistically limited and often unclear. Butler reports that Medicare regulations often hinder psychiatric care of the elderly.[5]

There are also severe limitations for physical and speech therapy under Medicare. Much effort is wasted because no home-care follow-up is provided after intensive rehabilitation work in the hospital.

The tangle of government bureaucracy or—in the case of supplementary insurance programs—private insurance company bureaucracy is oftentimes extremely frustrating. Regulations are constantly changing, and information given is often inconsistent and confusing. (If an elderly person is having trouble coping with Medicare, there's no reason to assume that it's *his* problem.)

Medicare benefits are constantly changing. New legislation concerning health care for the elderly is enacted regularly. Much of it concerns extended-care services. It is important to consider how these regulations and funding requirements directly determine the quality of care provided. As one experienced geriatric nurse declared, "Geriatrics is one-half money."

Categories of nursing homes are defined by their federal or state financing, but the category does not always describe the actual service given. There are two main categories of nursing homes: skilled nursing facilities and intermediate care facilities.

Skilled nursing facilities. There are two kinds of skilled nursing facilities. Extended-care facilities offer extended care beyond hospitalization for convalescence and rehabilitation. These facilities are not intended for long-term care. Skilled nursing care facilities are long-term, unlimited nursing homes, without the requirement of previous hospitalization and without necessarily requiring registered nurse care.

Intermediate care facilities. Personal care, simple medical care, and some nursing care are the services provided. These facilities are subject to federal rather than state regulations. Initially devised as cost-cutting facilities, they may, in some cases, cost more than skilled nursing care facilities for less care.

The regulations affect the quality of care in elaborate ways. Is physical therapy provided for in a particular institution? Dental care? Podiatry? Psychiatric care? Provisions may vary from state to state as well. Is the facility (and the regulations) suitable to the ideal care of the patient? Rarely, if ever. In fact, nurses learn how to make the best of what is available.

> I tried for 3 months to get a doctor to come in to check patients' teeth. *Everyone* needed something done—out of more than 50 patients the state turned everybody down.
>
> This decision was eventually reversed for some cases. Title 22 of Medicare provides for "oral hygiene." Any nurse can do oral hygiene. We need *dentistry.*[2]

Some states now provide long-term patients with monthly spending money. Nurses can help their patients spend it on anything from blank tape cassettes to monthly hair dressing. Most times, the money is not spent at all.

Restorative nursing, when it successfully restores a patient to greater independent living, is more economical than unneccessary long-term care. Ideally, restorative nursing methods could eventually rechannel enough money to make existing conditions closer to ideal.

Another government program that is just getting off the ground is in the area of homemaker or home-health-aid services. Home aides are provided by private agencies and, on a limited basis, public welfare programs. The cost of an adequate homemaker or home-aide service for the nation would not be cheap, but it would be a fraction of the expense of institutionalization. Home aides can be extremely valuable in many unforeseen ways. One aide, hired by a county agency to clean house for an elderly house-bound man for 4 hours a week, was able—in those few hours—to make his dark, dank home much more pleasant and enlivening, and provide companionship and conversation at the same time. The man's condition improved noticeably within 2 weeks. Unable to do his own housework, this man benefited *immensely* from clean, pleasant living space.

A final word about government programs—Medicare and Medicaid legislation have made the care of the elderly a potentially profitable business. The number of nursing homes more than doubled in the last decade; about 90% of these are profit-making. The United States is one of the few countries in the world in which the care of the sick and aged is "big business." Many nations in the world are able to provide total quality health care for the aged at no cost. We are not a leading nation in this regard. Our new knowledge about who the elderly are and what health services they require has forced us to look at our attitudes and the economic structure in an attempt to improve our approaches to geriatric nursing.

REFERENCES

[1]Karbach, E.: SAGE, Berkeley, Calif., 1975.

[2]Tyberg, D.: San Rafael, Calif. Interview, Dec. 11, 1975.

[3]Beauvoir, Simone de: *The Coming of Age.* New York: Putnam, 1972.

[4]Busse, E.W., and Pfeiffer, E.: *Mental Illness in Later Life.* Washington, D.C.: American Psychiatric Association, 1973.

[5]Butler, R.N., and Lewis, M.I.: *Aging and Mental Health.* St. Louis: C.V. Mosby, 1973.

SUGGESTED READING

David, H.M.: *Guidelines for Discharge Planning.* Downey, Calif.: Rancho Las Amigas, 1968.

Reiter, F.: "The Nurse Clinician." In *The Clinical Nurse Specialist.* Edited by E.P. Lewis. New York: American Journal of Nursing Co., 1970.

Appendix

Theories of Aging

EXTERNAL FACTORS IN AGING

The theories of individual aging that focus on external factors now emphasize four important areas of influence.

Environment

It has been well established that numerous environmental factors affect both health and life expectancy. These include air pollution, smoking, driving habits, and emotional pressures of all kind. Statistics indicate that a married man who lives in the country and who doesn't smoke can expect to live an impressive 22 years longer than a city bachelor who smokes two packs a day.

Nutrition

The significant influence of nutrition on life expectancy is well publicized. Experiments with mice demonstrate that mice fed high-fat diets become sick and appear extremely old while their littermates, fed on significantly less, remain healthy and active. Groups in which people reportedly reach very old age are also characterized by low-calorie diets, with little or no animal fat. Nutrition has an important, though little understood, relation to aging.

Bacteria and Viruses

These agents of disease also affect longevity. Some researchers suggest that nonpathogenic flora in the body may accelerate the aging process. Some viruses may be involved in physiological changes associated with normal aging.

Radiation

Although studies thus far have not confirmed that radiation plays a major role in aging, either directly or by inducing mutation, more research in this field is needed and is now underway.

These are the four major areas of concern with respect to external factors. Other theories focus on internal explanations for aging. Some suggest causes that are intrinsic to the body—that is, built into the system, and others postulate causes that are essentially malfunctions of the system.

MALFUNCTION THEORIES

There are two chief malfunction type theories. The first simply postulates that wear and tear are responsible for aging; the body, through loss of cells and decreased efficiency of the remaining cells, wears out.

The second malfunction theory is concerned with the accumulation of uncontrolled or random chemical reactions leading to disorder or structural change. Simply stated, research has found that such chemical reactions sometimes cause strong bonds between cells which are normally separate. This phenomenon, known as cross-linkage, may affect the functional capacity of the cells involved. Certain compounds, called free radicals because they contain an unpaired electron, are particularly prone to random reactions of this kind; this theory is often referred to as the free radical theory. When cell membranes are damaged by cross-linkage, they produce a residue stored in the cell, which has been identified as lipofuscin, or age pigment. The accumulation of this age pigment is a characteristic of aging.

As yet, lipofuscin has not been related to any functional decline. It has been discovered, however, that antioxidants, such as vitamin E, scavenge free radicals and thus prevent random reactions. It is possible that such therapy may eventually prove useful, but as yet it is not clear whether this process is a cause of aging, or one of its effects.

THEORIES ON INTRINSIC CAUSES

Finally, we come to the largest class of theories—those postulating an intrinsic cause of aging. Most scientists believe that aging is a built-in mechanism of some kind. One of these theories propounds a direct genetic program so that each individual inherits a particular life expectancy tendency. Another idea is that aging is the final consequence of development; An individual who remains immature for a longer period would expect to live longer.

A third theory suggest that certain genes have the specific function of causing mutations in other genes, and that these mutations play some role in the life expectancy of the individual. A fourth suggests that the accumulation of errors in all functions are responsible for eventual aging. Studies are also presently exploring the roles of enzymes and the genetic material within cell nuclei in the aging process. This list of possibilities reveals the wide scope of present research, as well as the fact that little is really known about the causes of aging.

OTHER THEORIES

Two other theories deserve special mention. Both approach aging from a higher biological level; rather than exploring the process in terms of cellular activity, these two are concerned with a more general process.

The immunologic theory of aging postulates that a gradual immunogenetic diversification of aging cells leads to a loss of recognition patterns between cells. This results in autoimmune reactions. This diversification may result from mutations, or the autoimmune reactions may be caused by a breakdown of homeostatic control of immune reactions. This is noteworthy since we have seen earlier that homeostatic control is generally weaker in old age.

Several conditions characteristic of various autoimmune diseases are associated with normal aging. These include rheumatoid factors, digestive conditions, and common blood conditions. Much experimentation has been devoted to this idea; one interesting series done with rats involved severe underfeeding for half the rats' lives. Longevity greatly increased, and this theory postulates that underfeeding may have suppressed immunologic development, since such important immunological sites as the spleen, liver, and gastrointestinal tract were most seriously affected.

The other higher level theory suggests that cells have a limited capacity to divide. Data indicates that old cells divide less often than young cells, when free of cancer. Cells, themselves, may have a limited life expectancy.

ADDITIONAL READING

This book is only an introduction to the field of geriatric nursing. More comprehensive literature is available, and may be very useful to the practitioner.

Books on Aging

Burnside, I.M.: *Nursing and the Aged.* New York, McGraw-Hill, 1976.

Burnside, I.M.: *Psycho-Social Nursing Care of the Aged.* New York, McGraw-Hill, 1973.

Butler, R.N.: *Why Survive? Being Old in America.* New York, Harper & Row, 1975.

Kimmel, D.C.: *Adulthood and Aging.* New York, John Wiley & Sons, 1974.

Kubler-Ross E.: *Death: The Final Stage of Growth.* Englewood Cliffs, New Jersey, Prentice-Hall, Inc., 1975.

Neugarten, B.L., (Ed): *Middle Age and Aging.* Chicago, University of Chicago Press, 1968.

Woodruff, D.S. and Birren J.E., (Eds): *Aging.* New York, Van Nostrand Reinhold Company, 1975.

Schoenberg, B., Garber, I., Wiener, A., Kutscher, A.H., Peretz, D., and Carr, A.C.: *Bereavement Its Psychosocial Aspects.* New York, Columbia University Press, 1975.

Journals on Aging and Related Subjects

American Journal of Nursing, American Nurses Association, 10 Columbus Circle, New York, N.Y. 10019.

Dynamic Maturity, American Association of Retired Persons, 1909 K St. N.W., Washington, D.C. 20036.

The Gerontologist, Gerontological Society, 1 Dupont Circle, Suite #520, Washington, D.C. 20036.

Journal of the American Geriatric Society, American Geriatric Society, 10 Columbus Circle, New York, N.Y. 10019.

Journal of Gerontology, Gerontological Society, 1 Dupont Circle, Suite #520, Washington, D.C. 20036.

Journal of Gerontological Nursing, Charles B. Slack, Inc. 6900 Grove Road, Thorofare, New Jersey 08086.

Journal of Social Issues, Society for the Psychological Study of Social Issues, Box 1248, Ann Arbor, Mich. 48106.

Fiction and Related Nonfiction

De Beauvoir, S.: *Coming of Age.* New York: G.P. Putnam's Sons, 1972. *A Very Easy Death.* New York: Warner Press, Inc., 1973.

Farrell, B.: *Pat and Roald.* New York: Random House, 1969.

Sarton, M.: *As We Are Now.* New York: W.W. Norton & Company Inc., 1973.

Townsend, C.: *Old Age: The Last Segregation.* Ralph Nader Study Group Report, New York: Grossman Publishers, 1971.

Wallant, E.L.: *The Human Season.* New York: Harcourt Brace Jovanovich, Inc., 1960.